BUS

BARCODE ON
NEXT PAGE

FIGHTING FAT!

Also by Kathleen Mayes

THE SODIUM-WATCHER'S GUIDE:
Easy Ways to Cut Salt and Sodium

OSTEOPOROSIS: Brittle Bones and The Calcium Crisis

OVERCOMING INDIGESTION

SUGAR: The Sweet Menace
(in preparation)

FIGHTING FAT!

How to Beat Heart Disease
and Cancer,
and Lose Weight

A Practical Guide to Fats, Oils and Cholesterol

Kathleen Mayes

Pennant Books, Santa Barbara, California

Pennant Books
3463 State Street, Suite 238
Santa Barbara, California 93105
U.S.A.

Library of Congress Cataloging-in-Publication Data

Mayes, Kathleen
    Fighting Fat! : how to beat heart disease and cancer,
    and lose weight / Kathleen Mayes.
        p.   cm.
    Bibliography: p.
    Includes index.
    ISBN 0-915201-28-3 ; ISBN 0-915201-29-1 (pbk.)
    1. Low-fat diet. 2. Food Fat content – health aspects.
3. Nutritionally induced diseases – Prevention – I. Title.
RM237.7.M39 1989
613.2'5--dc19   88-36469
                                                      CIP

Acknowledgments

Many national and international companies, organizations and government departments gave me invaluable material, cooperation and encouragement to produce this work. I particularly want to thank:

American Cancer Society
American Dietetic Association
American Heart Association
California Dietetic Association
Calorie Control Council
Cancer Information Service of California
Dairy Council of California
Department of Health and Social Security
Health Education Council
Institute of Shortening and Edible Oils, Inc.
International Olive Oil Council
Meat and Livestock Commission
Ministry of Agriculture, Fisheries and Food
National Cancer Institute
National Cattlemen's Association
National Dairy Council
National Heart, Lung and Blood Institute
National Institutes of Health
Norway Sardine Industry
Safflower Oil Information Bureau
Unilever PLC
U.S. Department of Agriculture

5

Author's Note

The use of any brand names in this guide is for identification only and does not imply endorsement or otherwise by the author. The author wishes to emphasize that the contents are intended to inform readers, but are not intended to replace the advice of physicians for individual ailments. Before beginning any significant changes in diet or usual amount of exercise, or undertaking any weight-loss program, readers are recommended to consult their doctor or professional health adviser.

Values for calories and fats have generally been obtained from U.S. Department of Agriculture Bulletin Number 72 *Nutritive Value of Foods*, revised 1985.

Foreword

Finally, a resource about dietary fat that describes how it is connected to heart disease, cancer *and* weight control! People are frequently confused by the mixed messages they receive about diet and disease. After reading *FIGHTING FAT!* readers will understand the disease processes and have more information to reduce their risk of these degenerative diseases as well as to interpret other information. The message that comes across in this book is obvious – a balanced diet is essential for everyone.

In addition to explaining the development of disease, readers will also gain knowledge on how to implement the recommended guidelines to reduce risk and help prevent disease. The practical application of the nutrition information is explained in detail. The author does an excellent job of teaching readers about the new ways of cooking and eating. She takes you through the process of revising recipes, with simple as well as more advanced ideas and suggestions. Mrs. Mayes knows her subject well; her enthusiasm for helping people change their diet is quite evident. *FIGHTING FAT!* makes readers *want* to change their diet, not only because of the benefits but because it is challenging and fun!

As a dietitian, I found the information very thorough and accurate. Any reader will appreciate this nutrition book because the information is very clear and concise. The charts and graphs that accompany the book are very helpful in summarizing the written information. The appendices give supplemental information that will be appreciated by all who use it.

Gerri French, M.S., R.D.
Registered Dietitian
Food For Fitness
Santa Barbara, CA

Contents

Introduction

Fat is an enemy. Its victims are everywhere.

A father of three youngsters dies suddenly of a heart attack at the age of 45. A favorite uncle is permanently crippled by a stroke. A top business executive has his leg amputated because of gangrene. A famous actress is stricken at the peak of her career by cancer of the breast. And the doctor has just told your best friend she is overweight and diabetic. Every day, people who think they are healthy suddenly discover they have a disease that ultimately disables or kills them.

By the year 2000, living to the age of 90 or 100 may be commonplace. But by adding to our life span, these extra years bring degenerative problems. Some of the most serious degenerative diseases of our time can be attributed to the high proportion of fat in our food supply.

It is no longer a proud boast that the average person in this country is "living off the fat of the land." More appropriate is the old saying "We are digging our graves with our forks." According to the *Surgeon-General's Report on Nutrition and Health, 1988,* the fat content of the average American's diet is 37 percent — estimates suggest some families have as much as 40 to 45 percent of their calories from fat. The American Heart Association, the National Cancer Institute and the American Cancer Society have all recommended that total fat intake be limited to *30 percent.*

The result of this disproportionate amount of dietary fat is a promotion of diseases that, taken together, account for over *half* the deaths in this country. News bulletins are full of grim statistics of sudden fatal accidents, especially auto accidents and deaths by homicide, but far outnumbering these deaths every day are those from cardiovascular causes and cancer. Roughly you stand a 50 percent chance of dying from heart disease. **FAT IS A KILLER – A 20th CENTURY PLAGUE!**

Too much fat in the diet can be responsible for cardiovascular diseases, the acceleration of the development of certain cancers, diabetes, and unneeded, unhealthy body fat. You cannot continue eating quantities of high fat foods and expect to remain fit. Many great scourges in history such as smallpox, typhoid and diphtheria have been eliminated or controlled by *prevention* – by an intervention before the onset of disease, rather than treatment or curing after the disease has been established. Similarly, we have solved the problem of acute food poisoning – but *not* the chronic poisoning that builds up over a period of time and leads to heart disease, high blood pressure and the promotion of cancers. While no microbes or viruses lurk behind the scenes in a heart attack, many problems associated with fat can, by and large, be anticipated, forestalled and prevented. Fats in large proportions are unnecessary and unhealthy, whereas a balanced diet in relation to fat can be good insurance to avoid many life-threatening, life-curtailing diseases.

Does good nutrition extend a person's life span? Does proper diet delay or prevent degenerative conditions such as atherosclerosis? To quote Dr. Jeffrey Blumberg, Associate Director of the Tufts University Nutrition Research Center (officially the U.S. Department of Agriculture Human Nutrition Research Center on Aging) in Boston, MA: "We're sure that nutrition is a major player in the aging process. . . .We think the day will come when we will be able to understand people's genes, and their nutritional needs, and put together a program that would give them long life."

A low-fat regimen can be preventive medicine, improving your chances of surviving to a ripe old age, enjoying good health without major surgery and large drug doses. *You* can do it.

1

From Stone Age
To Supermarkets

Mankind has survived successfully because intelligence helped humans to be opportunists, feeding on whatever was available to fill empty stomachs: plant material, animals, fish, insects – even clay, at times.

It seems to be natural to have a taste for fat, just as we have for sweet things, probably because our primate ancestors found it a rare treat to eat foods with these nutrients for millions of years. The diet of present-day baboons, chimpanzees and other primates reflects our more immediate prehuman ancestors. The genes of humans and chimpanzees differ by only about 1.5 per cent, even though our forebears diverged from theirs about 7 million years ago.

HOW MUCH HAVE WE CHANGED?
Over the hundreds of thousands of years that our bodies were evolving, our diet was being defined and it was largely vegetarian. So if there is a diet natural to our human makeup, one to which our genes and our digestive systems are still best suited, this is it.

Today's high-fat diet is out of harmony with human digestive and metabolic processes that our bodies have had for thousands of years. The human system is simply not made to handle a big fat intake. The amount and type of fat typically consumed in the Western diet represents a derangement of basic biological processes — a deviation from the pathways of metabolism that evolution has maintained and that are functionally similar to those of vertebrates generally. Most of the concentrations of oils and fats derived from grains and vegetables are recent inventions compared to the length of time the human body has taken to evolve. Our genes have not had time to adapt in any significant way to this particular challenge of fat consumption. The relatively new but widespread phenomenon of excessive fat intake over an entire life span is an overloading burden to the human system, incompatible with the biochemistry and physiology that have been predetermined by genetics.

COMPARATIVE PHYSIOLOGY
Compare the physiological characteristics of meat eaters (lions, tigers, dogs and cats) and fruit and vegetable eaters (monkeys, apes and chimpanzees, for instance). Humans are obviously closer to the latter:

Meat eaters:
Fangs for tearing flesh. No molars — chunks of meat are swallowed whole. Twenty times the hydrochloric acid in the stomach, compared with humans, to digest flesh quickly. Short intestinal tract to eliminate rapidly decaying waste products.

Fruit and vegetable eaters:
No sharp fangs. Well-developed molars for grinding vegetables and fruit, and enzymes in saliva to start digestion. Small amount of hydrochloric acid in stomach. Very long coiled intestinal tract to extract maximum amount from plant material that is slow to decay.

A major difference is found in the digestive tract. The relative length of the small intestine varies in different species: it is usually very long and coiled in herbivores, very short in carnivores, and of medium length in omnivores such as humans. High-fat foods are disastrous to the human system, which evolved to cope with light, low-fat vegetation (fruits, vegetables, legumes, roots, leaves, seeds and grains) high in carbohydrates and fiber. Almost all scientists and naturalists, including Charles Darwin, agree that the external and internal structure of humans is designed for fruits, grains and other high-fiber, high-carbohydrate vegetables.

THE HUMAN DIET IN PREHISTORY

While early humans may have relished fat in foods, under natural circumstances they would actually have eaten fat in only small amounts – nuts and seeds being mostly seasonal, wild game lean, small-yolked eggs from wild birds would have been relatively scarce, and the only milk was human, limited to the first few months of life. The hunting-foraging-gathering diet was eaten by all people on earth before the advent of agriculture 10,000 years ago. The Cro-Magnons in Europe between 35,000 and 10,000 years ago, used their simple weaponry with great skill in order to systematically exploit the large herds of game animals that roamed the scene. However, the relative proportions of animal and vegetable food consumed in the past can be ascertained by analyzing skeletal remains; bones contain both strontium (mostly found in plant foods) and calcium, so the bones of herbivores have a higher strontium/calcium ratio than those of carnivores. Analysis of this ratio in human fossils shows that the consumption of meat declined with the development of agriculture. Whether measured by weight or by calorie contribution, plants were the staple foods. Studies by pollen analysis and microscopic examination of husks, seeds and other plant remains have concluded that a wide variety of uncultivated vegetables, roots, wild fruits, berries, seeds and nuts were eaten, sometimes being brought to living sites from great distances.

Prehistoric peoples consumed mostly complex carbohydrates (unlike the refined sugars and finely-ground flours abundant in today's diet), with a greater intake of non-nutritive dietary fiber, and a higher proportion of potassium that far exceeded that of sodium (with the reverse now true among Westernized people around the world).

There was little smoking or drinking. Tobacco was non-existent in most of the Old World, although some pre-agricultural people in a few isolated locations and in certain seasons probably chewed tobacco. Alcohol (if preagricultural people had any indigenous brew) was probably only available seasonally, produced by natural fermentation and not dis-tillation, resulting in drinks such as beer of relatively low potency, and no spirits.

Life was short. Less than half the population lived to be twenty during Neanderthal times, and of the remaining adults, nine out of ten were dead before the age of forty. Many died from pneumonia; tuberculosis was widespread, and evidences of cancers and syphilis have been found. Many more must have been victims of diet-related diseases − of poisonous plants, contaminated food, seasonal malnutrition and severe vitamin deficiencies.

Sometime around 8000 B.C., Stone Age hunters were suc-ceeded by herders who grazed cattle, sheep and goats wherever pastures were good, and by farmers who scratched a living from the soil. Hitherto, deer had provided lean meat to hunting communities in Western Europe, but as farming cultures spread across the continent and improvements were made in cultivating crops, the food supply evolved to put even greater emphasis on grains and cereals. For centuries, peasants lived mainly on a thin gruel. In countries such as Greece, where land was too rocky to raise livestock, animal fats were scarce and in fact ancient Greeks and Romans disdained butter as mainly the food of barbarian cattle herders. They were beginning to produce oil from olives. Anatolia produced oil from almonds. On the other side of the globe, in Asia, oil came from soybeans and the coco-nut palm, while American Indians pressed oil from corn (maize).

WHAT DO YOU EAT – AND WHY?

Unlike animals of the same species who generally eat the same kind of food no matter where they live, humans are not controlled by strong instincts. We don't eat just for nourishment. We don't naturally crave the foods that we need or need the foods that we crave. There are a thousand factors involved in human eating. It is a pleasurable experience – enjoyable for most of us and a comfort for some. It is also a social experience. But why do you eat fat? Because you eat the meals you are *accustomed* to, from foodstuffs readily *available*. You eat the food you can *afford* – and that may not be the healthiest. How much fat you eat is generally determined by geography – where you were born, the cultural diet of that location, and the food habits of your family – and by social history, whether livestock animals were raised to be eaten or to provide beasts of burden. Food customs developed into thousands of cultures, following different guidelines from country to country, but basically evolved into three broad cultural diets:

Western, which is generally the Anglo-Saxon cultures of the United States, Britain and the Commonwealth, Europe and Russia. The early domestication of animals led to herding and dairying, and put the accent on meat and dairy products. The diet is *over 40 percent fat*.

Oriental, which is China, Japan, and other areas in the Far East. When Buddhism spread through Asia, it discouraged consumption of beef and other meats, made social outcasts of butchers, and fostered crop cultivation. With the emphasis on rice, vegetables and some fish, the diet is *about 10 percent fat*.

Developing or **Third World countries**, where people are either food gatherers or farmers of grains and vegetables that are directly consumed by the people rather than providing fodder for livestock. Very little meat is eaten because the people cannot afford it. *About 10 percent of the diet is fat*.

As a result, there are significantly large differences in health problems associated with each food culture. Epidemiological studies of cultures have shown that where diets contain only 10 to 12 percent fat calories, the rates for heart disease are negligible. For instance, Bantu natives in Africa living on fruits and leafy vegetables have almost no heart disease; but in the regions where British and Dutch settlers introduced cream, butter, cheese, meat and eggs, the heart disease rates are the same as in Europe.

On the other hand, Masai tribesmen drink a high-fat mixture of cows' milk and cows' blood, and studies reveal that their arteries become damaged. However, these people walk ten to twenty miles a day, and have developed blood vessels twice the size of an average European's — arteries large enough to deliver a full supply of blood and cause little heart disease.

RECENT HISTORY

Up to the beginning of this century, we obtained more calories from grains and vegetable sources. But as a country becomes wealthier, the cereal intake tends to decrease and the fat content to increase. Changes in diet can be traced to industrialization and the affluence it has given to more people to have a rich diet — literally to live "off the fat of the land." As we stopped growing our own produce and started shopping for food, in a sense we reverted to being hunter-gatherers, gathering whatever was available in the supermarkets.

The introduction of refrigeration and sophisticated processing made it possible to preserve, store and market fatty foods which, in earlier times, would have rapidly turned rancid. Technology enabled us to squeeze high concentrations of oils and fats from palm trees, seeds and nuts. The food industry began to exploit our preference for richer foods and our taste for fat, and the average worker has had a larger paycheck with more money to spend and the ability to afford to eat foods in any season that were formerly only available to the wealthy: meats, dairy products, white flour, white sugar.

The game our ancestors ate was lean, because most wild animals are unable to accumulate anything like the storage of fat found in layers under the skin or the marbling of muscle tissue found in today's domesticated meat. Even up to the 1850s, domesticated animals had usually been brought to market on the hoof, so that by the time the livestock reached the marketplace they were "lean and weary," lacking the thick saturated fat deposits we now expect them to have. The last few decades have seen the lean, stringy beef consumed by earlier agricultural societies transformed by selective breeding, restricted activity and altered feeding practices, the "finishing" of cattle at feedlots with energy-concentrated corn and grain. Feedlots have been fattening cattle for market, producing meat well streaked with fat because housewives wanted greater tenderness and were willing to pay for it. Cattle were forced into unnatural obesity by mankind's feeding systems. About the only food that humans have not tampered with is fish.

The growth of the dairy industry has been phenomenal. Before agriculture, people had no dairy foods at all except mother's milk, but the dairy farmer has been successful – too successful perhaps – in breeding and developing wild-ranging beasts into today's milk cows, highly-productive animals pampered in lush pastures, giving richer milk, creams, butters and cheeses with a higher butterfat content than ever before. As a result, the U.S. government has huge surpluses of cheese and butter, and the E.E.C. countries are faced with a butter mountain that is difficult to melt. Advertisers and marketing boards have been trying to induce us to use more cream and butter on or in food.

"Good food" has come to mean a lot of fat: breakfasts of bacon, eggs, flaky croissants and butter, coffee with cream; lunches of hamburgers, and French fries with everything . . . Nutritional problems of poor countries are those of scarcity. America's problems are caused by food abundance.

The next time you slather butter or margarine on a sandwich, or bite into a greasy hamburger, think how that fat will gum up your bloodstream, make a blood clot, deprive your heart of oxygen, or add a pound to your waist.

TABLE 1
PERCENTAGE OF CALORIES FROM FAT IN FOODS

Food Group	Less than 10%	10 to 20%	20 to 30%
Dairy products	nonfat milk, nonfat yogurt	buttermilk, lowfat cottage cheese	1% milk, lowfat yogurt, ice milk
Eggs	egg white		
Fats and oils	(none)	(none)	(none)
Fish and shellfish	canned shrimp, tuna canned in water	steamed scallops, baked sole	canned crab, broiled cod, raw oysters
Fruits	most fresh fruits and dried fruits		
Grains and cereals	bagels, grains, pastas, airpopped popcorn	breads, most breakfast cereals, most crackers, tortillas	bran muffins
Legumes, nuts, seeds	beans, peas, chestnuts		
Meats and meat products	(none)	(none)	dried chipped beef, lean roundsteak, venison
Mixed dishes and fast food	(none)	(none)	cheese pizza
Poultry and poultry products	(none)	roast chicken breast, roast turkey (light)	
Sugars and sweets	sugar, gumdrops, hard candies, jelly beans, jams, honey		caramel candies, chocolate fudge
Vegetables	all raw and steamed vegetables, baked potatoes		

TABLE 1 (*Continued*)

30 to 40%	40 to 50%	50 to 75%	More than 75%
2% milk, cottage cheese	whole milk, regular ice cream	goats milk, rich ice cream, Cheddar, Camembert, Swiss, ricotta, American processed cheese whole egg, eggnog	butter, whipping cream, sour cream, cream cheese
(none)	(none)	low-cal salad dressings	egg yolk margarine, mayonnaise, vegetable oils
tuna canned in oil, broiled halibut, fish-sticks, canned salmon	tuna salad, sardines in oil, breaded scallops, broiled trout, fried shrimp	pickled herrings, fried perch	
		avocados (Florida)	avocados (Calif.), coco-nuts, olives
granolas, apple pie, cakes, pancakes soybeans	croissants,Danish, cookies, donuts, popcorn in oil	bread stuffing, corn chips, cheesecake tofu	most nuts, peanut butter, sunflower seeds
eye of round, roast lamb leg, lamb loin, liver	Canadian bacon, canned ham, pork chop, corned beef, bottom round, veal, lamb rib	regular bacon, pork rib, beef rib roast, chuck roast, sirloin steak, pork links, dry salami	most cold cuts, frankfurters, brown & serve sausages
roast beef sandwich	macaroni & cheese, hamburger, chili con carne	cheeseburger, enchilada, fish sandwich, quiche	
roast turkey (dark)		duck, goose, fried chicken, chicken frankfurter	
fudge syrup	chocolate pudding, lemon curd spread	chocolate bars	baking choco-late
mashed potatoes, potatoes au gratin	French fries, scalloped potatoes, hash browns	potato chips, potato salad, fried onion rings	fried mush-rooms, cole-slaw

Avoiding fat can be a tricky business. You probably eat far more fat than you realize and far more fat than you need, because most fat is *concealed* (see Table 1).

Maybe only a third of the fat you consume is actually visible — such as the strips of hard fat on meats, the oils used in preparing food, and oil-based salad dressings. Fat is an integral part of hard cheese and cream cheese, cream soups, ice cream, cake frostings and nuts. The food industry has taken charge of our diet, using ingredients that include chemicals which are unfamiliar and unpronounceable. Do-it-yourself control has been exchanged for prepackaged convenience, with instant-this, powdered-that and imitation-the-other, ready-prepared for popping into boiling water or the microwave. Fat can be a major ingredient in many factory-prepared composite food products, such as:

- processed meats and sausages
- sardines and tuna-fish packed in oil
- pies, cakes, biscuits and cookies
- snack foods, nuts and potato chips
- breakfast mueslis and granolas
- artificial "whiteners" and "creamers" for coffee and tea.

Think of the menus in restaurants where there is an overabundance of dishes which are:

- au gratin, au fromage, or in a cheese sauce
- buttery, buttered, or in a butter sauce
- au lait, or à la mode
- creamed, or in a cream sauce
- in a Hollandaise sauce
- topped with sour cream.

Fast-food chains have grown and prospered on fried foods, which multiply the fat content of a basic food item. Examples: French fries have more than eighty times the fat of baked potatoes; fried shrimp have more than ten times the fat of boiled shrimp; a mere 2 ounces (56g) of potato chips can have the equivalent of 4 teaspoons (20ml) of fat.

Children now eat these high-fat foods from their youngest days, so that their tastes are shaped to prefer and expect such food, with their arteries getting an early start at becoming clogged.

Supermarkets are full of processed food products, with compounds sometimes only recognizable by a chemist, but fat is one of the principal ingredients.

Why are fats heavily used? The answer is simple: fats are cheap. Supermarkets are jungles, with customers often enticed by the jangle of advertising for the hundreds of new food items — but the food manufacturers listen only for the jingle at the cash registers. Food processing is big business, with unhealthy fat being the most profitable. Food processors choose ingredients that travel well and cheaply, have a long shelf life, and are least likely to turn rancid — the fats that are solid and stable at room temperature. On supermarket shelves you find many basic foods that are now made into pastries, prepared mixes, snack foods, frozen dinners and other items with a much higher fat content, or are garnished with butter, cream or salad dressing.

Even if you are trying to follow what is supposed to be a more healthful diet by rejecting red meat, you may be replacing it with fattier foods. For example, nuts, seeds and nut butters; quiches with fat in the cheese, in the cream, and in the pie-crust; or salads featuring whole avocados and heavy dressings. In some nuts, 85 percent of the calories are fat calories, and a half-cup of nuts has the equivalent of 5 teaspoons (25ml) of fat. In avocados and sunflower seeds, 75 percent of the calories are fat calories. Even innocuous-looking apples are coated with waxy oil substances to reduce moisture loss during shipping.

We have gone from a culture of poverty to a food feast made up of dangerous foods, high in various animal fats and cholesterol. Arteries are becoming clogged with these fat compounds, and overweight is a problem because greasy foods have high concentrations of calories. Heart disease, hardening of the arteries, and too much body fat are not just problems for the elderly, but are becoming more prevalent each year in younger and younger children.

Fat is indispensable to our diets, and to eliminate it completely would be harmful. Fats have components that our bodies cannot synthesize from other dietary sources. But the amounts of fat you eat, and the kinds of fat you choose, can ruin your health and shorten your life span.

This is not to suggest that the ancient hunting-gathering societies were healthier than our own. They often suffered early death from infections and diseases that we can now control. But by picking and choosing the best from their lifestyle along with the best from ours, we should be able to forestall or even prevent many of the currently prominent diseases and thereby live longer, healthier lives. **One prudent step is to cut fat.**

2

What Are Fats?

Fat is a nasty word in the minds of many people. To them, it means being overweight or obese, something to avoid. So why do you need it? It is easy to forget, or ignore, the fact that the body does need some fat in the diet for good health. Virtually all living forms require some type of fat. Despite its bad press, fat is essential for life, and is a basic food nutrient:

* It makes food more palatable.
* It gives a feeling of satisfaction and fullness after a meal.
* It supplies essential fatty acids.
* It is a source of fuel and energy.
* It protects vital organs and nerves.
* It helps to transport certain vitamins around your body.

Fat plays an important role in the stimulation of saliva. Much of the taste and texture in foods comes from fat, making foods more palatable, more tender and enjoyable.

Eating a meal containing fat can give you a sense of fullness and satisfaction, as the fat sends signals to your stomach to turn off the gastric juices that aid digestion. Fats are absorbed by the intestines over a period of up to six hours – far slower than proteins or carbohydrates – so fats help to reduce the feeling of hunger between meals.

Fat in food provides essential fatty acids, including *linoleic and linolenic acid*, which are of major importance to health. They are termed essential because your body is unable to produce them, or cannot make them in sufficient amounts, so they have to be supplied by the food you eat. Linoleic acid is especially necessary for proper growth in children. It is needed to perform various roles in metabolism, including the maintenance of cell membranes, regulating cholesterol metabolism, and helping to create *prostaglandins* (hormone-like substances needed for several body processes), and maintaining a healthy skin, preventing drying and flaking.

Fat is a body fuel, with the burning of fat in your body just as wood is burned in a fire; as a stockpile and source of fuel it maintains your body warmth. Fat, like carbohydrates, proteins and alcohol, is a source of energy and calories, with fat providing nine calories for every gram — a greater concentration than from protein or carbohydrates which provide only four calories per gram. If you eat more fat than your body needs at any one time, it stores it in various depots: usually half is stored beneath the skin, helping the synthesis of sunshine into a pre-vitamin D, with the remaining fat being confined to the trunk and little at the lower extremities. Fat layers under the skin, your fuel reserves, are a most efficient insulation against body-heat loss — obese people can be most uncomfortable in hot weather, but in a cold climate they can conserve body heat and remain warm while lean people are shivering.

A limited amount of fat on your body serves as a protection for vital organs, providing cushions around kidneys, stomach and intestines, to protect them from physical shock. The liver can store about four percent of its weight in fat. Nerves are also covered with a fat material called the *myelin sheath*. This sheath may serve as a protection for the nerve trunk and as an insulation similar to the covering on an electric wire. A newborn's nervous system does not have a complete myelin covering, which suggests that the nerves cannot function perfectly until fully insulated. Consequently, a small child's heat-regulating system is not very effective until myelinization is complete.

When you eat fat, it acts as a carrier for vitamins into your body. Generally speaking, most fats and oils are not good sources of vitamins other than vitamin E, but fat-soluble vitamins A, D and K can only be transported into your system and absorbed through the intestinal wall by way of fat (which is why food manufacturers fortify margarines with vitamins A and D), giving fat an important function in proper nutrition.

HOW MUCH (OR HOW LITTLE) DO YOU NEED?
A diet severely deficient in fat can harm the efficiency of gland function. Fat-soluble vitamins cannot be conveyed and absorbed into your system. Sebaceous glands that produce lubricants can be affected, causing dryness of skin and scalp. There may also be a decrease in joint lubrication.

When babies are fed skimmed milk and raw vegetables rather than the high-energy foods they need, health-conscious parents are inadvertently starving infants. By trying to avoid obesity or development of heart disease, they produce an undernourishment which retards growth and development of their babies to such an extent that they have a low risk of survival similar to premature or low birth-weight babies.

But when you are an adult, only a small amount of essential fatty acids are needed by your body. About one to two percent of your day's calories should contain linoleic acid, so a tablespoon of corn oil, for example, provides more linoleic acid than is needed by most people. However, nutritionists think it unwise to try to limit essential fatty acid intake to such a tiny amount. The Pritikin eating program provides only ten percent of total calories from fats. Even when severe fat-restricted diets or weight reduction plans are prescribed, most nutrition experts believe, however, that about 20 percent of calories should come from fats. Meals extremely low in fat would be dull, leaving you hungry soon after eating.

Few people in this country suffer from nutritional deficiencies because they eat too little fat, but many obviously suffer from overconsumption.

HOW MUCH IS TOO MUCH?

Most nutrition and health experts agree that Americans eat too much fat. We have one of the highest fat-containing diets in the world, with fat intake in some families rising to as much as 40 or 45 percent of total calories consumed. This increase is attributed mainly to the fact that many people are eating more processed foods and fast foods containing a high percentage of grease, fat or oil — and they are eating more meat and cheese than years ago. Leading health authorities would like to see fat consumption modified to no more than *30 percent* of daily calories. So if, typically, you eat food with roughly 2,000 calories a day, no more than 600 calories should be from fat, that is 67 grams or 2 1/2 ounces. Of that 30 percent, no more than 10 percent should be *saturated*, a term explained later in this chapter.

WHAT IS FAT?

To a chemist, fats and oils are predominantly mixtures of fatty acids and glycerol commonly called *triglycerides*. Triglycerides belong in a group referred to as *lipids*. In 100 grams of fat, 95 grams will be triglycerides; the other 5 grams will include mono-glycerides, diglycerides, phosphatides (such as lecithin), sterols (such as cholesterol), tocopherols (that retard rancidity and provide a source of vitamin E), carotenoids (that give fat its natural yellowish tinge) and other trace substances.

WHAT HAPPENS TO FATS IN YOUR SYSTEM?

Before you put that bite of fat into your mouth with a fork, think about what is going to happen to it. In your mouth the food is mixed and moistened with your saliva and then mechanically broken down into smaller pieces by chewing. After swallowing, the fat passes down the esophagus, or gullet, into your stomach where it is mixed with gastric juice, and contractions cause further mechanical breakdown. Foods high in fat can remain in the stomach for four to six hours, unlike carbohydrates which can pass through in as little as two hours. The exact time in your stomach can depend on your emotional state.

Most digestion and absorption occurs in the 22 to 25 feet (6.7 to 7.6 meters) of small intestine, first in the duodenum section, then in the jejunum and finally the ileum. In the duodenum the food mixture is attacked by digestive juices — bile, pancreatic juice and intestinal juice. Bile salts, produced by the liver and stored in the gallbladder, break the fat into minute droplets; *lipase* enzymes from the pancreas and intestinal wall split the triglyceride molecules into fatty acid units and glycerol. The fatty acids are then absorbed through the wall of the intestine along with fat-soluble vitamins. After passing through the intestinal lining, most fat is re-formed into triglycerides and emptied into the bloodstream; they are now known as *serum triglycerides*.

In the bloodstream, the plot thickens, as it were . . .

Fat is moved from place to place via the bloodstream, and any tissue that needs fat must get it from the blood. Although fat is generally insoluble in water, it moves freely in the watery medium of blood and tissues: the microscopic particles of fat have to attach themselves temporarily to a protein molecule, with the combination then known as a *lipoprotein*.

Lipoproteins include chylomicrons, very low-density lipoproteins (VLDL), low-density lipoproteins (LDL) and high-density lipoproteins (HDL). The lipoproteins differ from each other in chemical composition, in size and their function in the body. The chief conveyers of triglycerides in your blood are the relatively large chylomicrons and the smaller VLDLs. If you could see your blood after you have eaten a fatty meal, it would look temporarily turbid and cloudy; chylomicrons, formed in the intestine, and the small VLDLs made in the liver and small intestine, are transporting triglycerides through your bloodstream. A couple of hours later, your blood clears as the chylomicrons leave the bloodstream and the microscopic fat particles are absorbed into your adipose tissue (fat stores) or to the liver for immediate use. The VLDLs are broken down by enzymes to form the LDLs. The LDLs are the chief transporters of cholesterol, they can deposit cholesterol in the linings of blood vessels and are major culprits in the development of atherosclerosis — the villains associated with heart problems.

The very small HDL molecules, on the other hand, transport excess cholesterol from blood vessels and out of your body, acting like an arterial "Drano." Women, before menopause, have more of the desirable HDLs in their bloodstream and as a consequence have about one-third the chance of developing heart disease compared to men of the same age. The level of LDL should be no more than 160 milligrams per deciliter of blood; if you have other risk factors, your LDL should be 130 to 160 mg/dl. A normal HDL level is 45 mg/dl or

---

THE ROLE OF CHOLESTEROL

Everyone by now must have heard the word "cholesterol", probably in a fragmentary way. But just what is it? Pure cholesterol is an odorless, white, powdery substance found in all foods of animal origin and is part of every animal cell, including fish and chicken and particularly organ meats and egg yolks. It is not found in fruits and vegetables.

Cholesterol is not a type of fat but a close associate known as a sterol, a fat-like substance. Dietary cholesterol is not visible to the eye and you cannot taste it in the foods you eat, but your body uses it to make cell walls and nerve tissue; the sex glands and adrenal glands use cholesterol to make certain hormones. The liver also converts cholesterol into bile acids that are needed for complete food digestion. Even if you didn't eat any cholesterol, your liver manufactures enough for your body's needs — between 500 and 1,000mg a day — and after the first six months of life you don't actually need any more than you manufacture. As the body absorbs cholesterol after eating, the liver tries to ratchet down its cholesterol output, but it isn't always an even exchange, and cholesterol levels can rise quickly. Blood or serum cholesterol and plasma cholesterol all refer to the same thing: the cholesterol that is circulating in your blood. Blood cholesterol contains both the cholesterol coming from your diet and that made by your liver.

---

greater. A ratio of at least 3 to 1 is considered desirable. Studies show that if you exercise, do not smoke and have a reasonable body weight, you can increase the ratio of HDLs in your bloodstream.

Further changes in fats may be made by your body in its metabolism, either burning them for energy needs, storing them in adipose layers as a reserve for future energy needs, or synthesizing prostaglandins and thromboxanes which regulate various body processes.

Cholesterol is similar to a fat in that it will not mix with water, so in order to be carried in the bloodstream, it becomes bonded, like fat, to proteins in lipoprotein bundles, and can be found in both LDLs and HDLs.

The average American derives between 350 and 450mg of cholesterol each day from diet (sometimes as much as 530mg), a Frenchman just less than 500mg, but a Japanese only about 130mg. In the typical Western diet, serum cholesterol is raised mostly by eating saturated fat, although the cholesterol in other foods also contributes. A food such as an egg may contain only a moderate amount of saturated fat but substantial cholesterol. The amount of cholesterol absorbed from the diet can vary between 20 and 50 percent, depending on how much fat you eat and the kind of fat. Once cells have taken in cholesterol, they dispose of it very slowly. Polyunsaturated fats will lower blood cholesterol, but only half as much as saturated fats will raise it.

According to the National Heart, Lung and Blood Institute, it is usual for cholesterol levels to be slightly higher in winter and lower in summer, where climate changes are considerable. No one can yet explain the seasonal change, beyond speculating that people tend to eat more meats and fatty foods in winter, whereas during summertime they have more fruits and vegetables.

Feces (body wastes) normally contain from 5 to 25 percent of fatty material including free fatty acids and sterols. Fats are present even if you are on a fat-free diet. About one-third of fecal lipids consists of sterols, mainly cholesterol. If you have a deficiency of pancreatic lipase or bile salts, fat not completely digested will be excreted. An excess of fat in the stool, *steatorrhea*, is a symptom in a number of diseases, particularly *tropical sprue*, the defective digestion of fat. When sprue inhibits fat digestion, undigested fat in the intestine actually greases it, causing diarrhea (which is the way mineral oil acts as a laxative).

THE COMPOSITION OF FATS

If a fatty substance is solid at room temperature it is usually called a "fat" and typically includes butter, lard and beef fat. But if a dietary fat is liquid at room temperature, it is generally termed an "oil." Appendix I shows the most frequently used animal fats and vegetable oils coming from a wide range of sources: from various land animals, marine life, from plants, trees, seeds and nuts grown in all climates of the world, from the Tropics to the Poles. Whereas certain oils were formerly confined more or less to local areas where they were produced, they are now shipped to many other countries and regions to create a vast selection from which to choose.

Biochemists group dietary fat into *saturated, monounsaturated,* and *polyunsaturated* fatty acids (PUFAs) − terms which refer to the chemical structure of the fat molecules. Foods that contain fat usually have varying proportions from each group (see Table 2).

Saturated fat, hard at room temperature, is found mostly in meats and dairy products, for example beef suet, lard and butterfat.

Monounsaturated fat is found primarily in peanut (groundnut) and olive oils.

Polyunsaturated fat, usually soft or liquid at room temperature, is mostly in vegetable oils such as safflower, sunflower, corn, soybean and cottonseed, and in fish. Notable exceptions are tropical oils.

TABLE 2
TYPICAL FATTY ACID COMPOSITION OF THE
PRINCIPAL VEGETABLE OILS AND ANIMAL FATS

Oil or fat	Percentage of total fatty acids*		
	Saturated	Mono-unsaturated	Poly-unsaturated
Beef tallow	46	47	4
Butterfat	63-70	28-31	1-3
Canola (low erucic acid rapeseed) oil	6	62	32
Cocoa butter	61	34	3
Coconut oil	92	6	2
Corn oil	13	28	59
Cottonseed oil	26	20	55
Fish oil (menhaden)**	32	31	3
Lard	42	48	10
Margarine:			
Hard: All vegetable	18-21	45-66	14-35
Animal/vegetable	29-40	46-52	9-19
Soft: All vegetable	17-19	33-52	29-48
Spreads: All vegetable	17-20	32-54	27-50
Olive oil	17	72	11
Palm oil	50	40	10
Palm kernel oil	82	15	2
Peanut oil	14	50	32
Safflower oil	9	13	78
Shortening:			
All vegetable fat	24-30	43-65	10-30
Animal/veg. fat blend	40-49	46-51	4-11
Soybean oil	15	24	61
Sunflower oil	12	19	69

* Fatty acid composition may not add to 100 percent due to rounding.
** Menhaden oil also contains 21 percent omega-3 fatty acids.
(Adapted from *Food Fats and Oils*, January 1988. Reproduced with the kind permission of the Institute of Shortening and Edible Oils, Inc., Washington, D.C.)

For reasons not yet completely understood, plants growing in colder climates start out making saturated fat from glucose; they then convert it to more unsaturated forms, perhaps because saturated fats (which harden when the temperature drops low enough) would interfere with cellular functions. Plants growing in warmer climates, on the other hand, produce more saturated oils, so there are vegetable fats that are highly saturated (more so than animal fats), which include *coconut oil, palm oil* and *cocoa butter* (used in chocolate). These tropical oils are really similar to hard fats.

PROCESSING

All fats and oils go through several processes of extraction, refining, bleaching, deodorizing, and hydrogenation. Manufacturers may add government-approved additives (such as tocopherols, BHA and BHT) to protect quality during storage and shipping of the products. Some oils are "winterized" with the removal of crystallized fatty acids before bottling, to prevent clouding when they are refrigerated. Oils that are naturally liquid and mostly PUFA may undergo varying degrees of hydrogenation to make products that are more solid and stable, such as hard margarines and cooking fats, giving them a longer shelf life before they turn rancid. These resulting products are more saturated since hydrogenation adds hydrogen to change the molecular structure. The word "hydrogenated" on a label usually indicates a product that is high in saturates, although this may not always be the case as many degrees of hydrogenation are possible, and much depends on the original percentage of saturated fat before it undergoes this treatment. If a liquid oil is labeled "partially hydrogenated," the hydrogenation has been slight. Palm and coconut oils, however, are already naturally saturated, so the process of hydrogenation increases their saturated fat content from *high* to *higher.* The process has been criticized for creating an unnatural form of fat known as *trans fat* which has a slightly rearranged chemical structure.

FATS UNDER THE MICROSCOPE

Most fatty acids are straight chains of up to 24 carbon atoms and each of these may be linked to hydrogen atoms (see Figure 1).

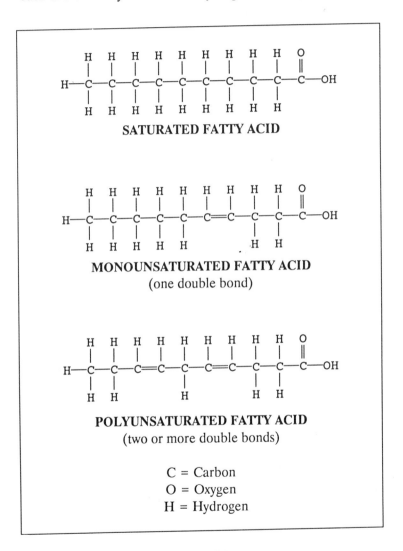

SATURATED FATTY ACID

MONOUNSATURATED FATTY ACID
(one double bond)

POLYUNSATURATED FATTY ACID
(two or more double bonds)

C = Carbon
O = Oxygen
H = Hydrogen

FIGURE 1
MOLECULAR STRUCTURES OF FATTY ACIDS

The number of carbon and hydrogen atoms in a fatty acid, along with the different combinations of fatty acids found in a particular fat, determines the type of fat it is and how it tastes. See Table 3 for the fatty acids which occur most frequently in foods.

Why do you need to know these minute details about fatty acids? Because the different fatty acids have various characteristics used by the body in different ways and they can determine how much dietary cholesterol you absorb or harmlessly excrete. Trans fats are suspected in the promotion of tumors. Saturated fats have the capacity to raise blood cholesterol, hence the recommendation to limit them to 10 percent of calories, whereas PUFAs and monounsaturates tend to reduce the amount of cholesterol in the blood and enhance its excretion. But large amounts of PUFAs may promote tumor growth and suppress your immune function. Some fats hasten the formation of blood clots; other oils encourage blood to flow smoothly (see Chapter 3).

The key point is that when shopping in the supermarket, cooking in the kitchen, choosing dishes in restaurants and fast-food chains, you are determining the quantity of fat and the type of fat you eat and put into your bloodstream. You are in fact making crucial decisions that may determine whether or not you ultimately develop high blood pressure, clog your arteries, have a heart attack or stroke, become vulnerable to cancer, add extra poundage, or increase your risk of diabetes and gallstone disease.

TABLE 3
COMMON NAMES OF FATTY ACIDS

Carbon atoms	Double bonds	Common name	Main sources
Saturated:			
4	0	Butyric	Butterfat
6	0	Caproic	Butterfat
8	0	Caprylic	Coconut oil
10	0	Capric	Coconut oil
12	0	Lauric	Coconut oil
14	0	Myristic	Butterfat, coconut oil
16	0	Palmitic	Most fats and oils
18	0	Stearic	Most fats and oils
20	0	Arachidic	Shortening, hard margarine, peanut oil
22	0	Behenic	Peanut oil
24	0	Lignoceric	Peanut oil
Monounsaturated:			
10	1	Caproleic	Butterfat
12	1	Lauroleic	Butterfat
14	1	Myristoleic	Butterfat
16	1	Palmitoleic	Fish oils, shortening, beef fat, lard, butter
18	1	Oleic	Most fats and oils, egg yolks
18	1	Elaidic	Butterfat, beef fat
18	1	Vaccenic	Butterfat, beef fat
20	1	Gadoleic	Some fish oils
22	1	Erucic	Rapeseed oil, shortening, hard margarine
Polyunsaturated:			
18	2	Linoleic	Most vegetable oils
18	3	Linolenic	Rapeseed oil, soybean oil, wheatgerm oil
20	4	Arachidonic	Shortening, lard
20	5	Eicosapentaenoic	Some fish oils
22	6	Docosahexaenoic	Some fish oils

(Adapted from *Food Fats and Oils*, January 1988. Reproduced with the kind permission of the Institute of Shortening and Edible Oils, Inc., Washington, D.C.)

3

Fats and Cardiovascular Disease

When actor Peter Sellers died at the age of fifty-four, the hospital spokesman said he died of "natural causes." But there is nothing *natural* about dying of heart disease at fifty-four. Heart muscle and blood vessels are meant to last a lot longer than that. The problem of clogged arteries is largely self-inflicted. Dr. Paul Dudley White, the eminent cardiologist, said "heart disease before eighty is our own fault, not God's or Nature's will."

In the United States, during the past twenty years, the death rate from coronary disease has dropped by 37 percent, but the problem is far from over. The Surgeon-General reports that heart disease is still the leading killer of Americans: more than 500,000 deaths as a result of 1.25 million heart attacks every year. In 1985, illness and death from heart disease cost Americans an estimated $49 billion in direct health care costs and lost productivity.

YOUR CARDIOVASCULAR SYSTEM
Your cardiovascular system is like a system of highways and byways with your bloodstream carrying all kinds of traffic

bearing loads of different nutrients to all parts of your body. Think of your circulatory system as having two halves — arterial and venous. Arteries carry blood away from the heart to the tissues; the largest artery is called the aorta and the smallest arteries are known as arterioles. To carry blood back to the heart, you have veins with the smallest known as venules. Connecting arterioles and venules are capillaries, the tiniest blood vessels which are so fine that red blood cells have to proceed in single file. Cells clumped together by fat and oil cannot get through. The exchange of waste materials, nutrients and gases within cells takes place as blood passes through capillaries. The busy highway system reaches all parts of your body and all organs, one of the most important being the liver, which serves as a warehouse monitoring your stocks of nutrients in the bloodstream.

Blood is both a tissue and a fluid. It is pumped through your body, playing a vital part in its functioning. It acts as a conveyor for nutrients, much like container trucks on the freeways. It is a tissue because it has a collection of cells, and these cells are suspended in a pale amber fluid called plasma. The total amount of blood circulating in the body varies with your age, sex, weight and body build, but a rough average for adults is 7 to 8 percent of body weight, equal to about 10 1/2 pints (5 liters). About 6 3/4 pints (3.2 liters) is plasma delivering nutrients, blood cells and waste products, and helping to maintain blood pressure and to distribute heat uniformly throughout the body. Plasma carries calcium, glucose, proteins, salts, hormones and lipoproteins carrying various cargoes of cholesterol and fat globules (lipids) originating from either the diet or the body's fat stores. The remaining 3 3/4 pints (1.8 liters) are millions of cells — cells so small that 60,000 would cover a pinhead: red cells containing hemoglobin which conveys oxygen to and carbon dioxide away from tissues; five types of white cells which are the body's ambulances rushing to hunt down and destroy infection; and platelets (thrombocytes) which enable the blood to clot.

Your blood's contents act as an important indicator of many things – how well you are eating, what you are eating and drinking, and if you are sick. You can do a great deal to get the right things into your blood and keep the wrong things out. The amount of oxygen the blood conveys can be an indicator of how much you are exercising – or smoking. To help your blood carry more oxygen, you can stop smoking and at the same time fight air pollution!

Blood pressure. As your heart pumps blood through the arteries, the push of this blood on the artery walls determines the amount of pressure. Artery walls are elastic, particularly in younger years; they stretch and contract to take the ups and downs of blood pressure. To measure pressure, many types of monitors are now available, with sphygmomanometers being the most usual (from Greek: *sphygmos* = pulse, *metron* = measure). You are probably familiar with the inflatable rubber cuff that your doctor places around your upper arm and inflates to restrict blood flow. Dr. N.C. Koratkoff first used this device in St. Petersburg (now Leningrad), Russia, in 1905, and the sounds your doctor hears in his stethoscope when taking blood pressure are still known as Koratkoff sounds. A pressure reading of 120/80 is considered normal. The numbers have their origins in the height in millimeters that your blood will force a column of mercury up a tube, although these days the device is likely to have a dial or an electronic digital readout. The pressure is measured at two moments during the heart-beat cycle: the first and highest of the two numbers is a measurement of the force of blood in the arteries as the heart contracts at the peak of the beating cycle (the phase called *systolic*). The second and lower of the two numbers is the force of blood in the vessels at the low point of the heart's contractions when your heart is relaxing and resting between beats in order to fill again with blood (the phase called *diastolic*). Another less frequently used but more accurate method to measure blood pressure involves inserting a catheter into an artery. The catheter is connected to an instrument that records the blood pressure as an electronic signal.

There is no blood-pressure reading that is "normal" for everyone. Your age, sex, and overall health help your doctor determine what is normal and healthy for you. Blood pressure not only varies among people but it can vary in the same person at different times: it is at its lowest during sleep, rising and varying during the day depending upon whether you are sitting or standing, having a cigarette, becoming excited or having sex. Even the stress of going to the doctor's office, fighting traffic along the way, may temporarily raise your blood pressure, which is why if you have a high reading the doctor may want to recheck it several times. Trouble begins when blood pressure goes up and stays up.

Hypertension. This refers to the condition of high pressure of blood in arteries – not to tension in the sense of stress or anxiety – although chronic anxiety can elevate blood pressure. It means that the force of the blood pressing against the walls of your arteries is above the normal range for your age. High pressure indicates that the arteries are either narrowed or tightened, and the heart has to work harder to pump blood. A major cause of hypertension is the accumulation of fats on the inside of arterial walls, causing resistance to blood flow. For people who are 18 years of age and older, use the following chart as a guide:

Systolic blood pressure (with a diastolic reading of less than 90):

Reading:	Category:
Less than 140	Normal blood pressure
140 to 159	Borderline isolated systolic hypertension
160 or more	Isolated systolic hypertension

Diastolic blood pressure:

Reading:	Category:
Less than 85	Normal blood pressure
85 to 89	High normal blood pressure
90 to 104	Mild hypertension
105 to 114	Moderate hypertension
115 or more	Severe hypertension

For adults, 140/90 is considered the borderline between normal and high. Children and teenagers should always have lower blood-pressure readings.

Your doctor is the best person to know whether you have high blood pressure, and readings are usually included in routine physical examinations, with results generally available if you ask for them. Home-kits are available to monitor your condition regularly without seeing your physician.

High blood pressure is such a stealthy condition, doing damage without symptoms before you even know you are suffering from it. In fact most of the damage goes on inside you − inside your arteries, inside your kidneys, even inside your eyes − where you cannot feel it. Most of the time there are few warning signs or symptoms although you may experience dizziness, headaches, tiredness or nosebleeds. Shortness of breath when you walk may be a sign of blood pressure out of control. If you are overweight and/or a heavy smoker, you run a greater risk of high blood pressure. Or you may be sensitive to excessive table salt, or the sodium in salt and other foods, which with defects in the kidneys or the adrenal cortex, can cause the blood to retain liquids. Regular exercise is helpful in bringing blood pressure down (excluding such activities as weight lifting which can be dangerous to hypertensives).

High blood pressure tends to run in families. In some people, the muscle cells of the arterioles, which carry blood from the larger arteries to the capillaries, tighten up and stay tightened, although why arterioles constrict abnormally is still subject to research.

The Arteries. Walls of the arteries consist of three layers: *adventitia*, *media* and *intima*. The adventitia is the tough, fibrous outermost layer that helps the arteries to maintain their cylindrical shape and provide support. The media is a firm band of interwoven elastic filaments and muscle fibers exerting a constant pressure to control the diameter of the blood vessel and thus the blood pressure of the column of blood within. The intima (or so-called lumen) is the innermost layer − a thin membrane or sheathing of flattened cells presenting what should be a smooth streamlined surface in contact with the blood flowing through the vessel (see Figure 2a).

When blood pressure is high, it affects the circulation throughout the body, but seems to cause the most damage to the delicate inner lining of the coronary arteries, especially where they branch into smaller channels. Old anatomy texts used to compare the diameter of coronary arteries to that of a quill pen; newer comparisons suggest that of a drinking straw, with the channels being about 1/8 inch (3mm) wide.

Fatty streaks in the neighborhood of the adventitia and media layers of artery walls are apparently harmless, but when deposits are present in the intima they can protrude into the passageway of the vessel and are known as *atheromatous plaques* (see Figures 2b and 2c).

Although considered a plague of the twentieth century, atherosclerosis is not new: in 1973, doctors at Wayne State University, Detroit, performed an autopsy on a mummified man who had died 2,100 years ago in Ancient Egypt. This aristocrat of ancient times, although only aged between 35 and 40 years at his death, had "large and small plaques in portions of the aorta."

In 1755, Dr. Albrecht von Haller, a Swiss physician, described the softenings that occur on artery walls as resembling gruel, from which he labeled the softening *atheroma* (from two Greek words: *athera* = gruel and *oma* = tumor). In 1904 a French physician coined the term *atherosclerosis*. In 1910 the greasy crystalline substance that looked like gruel to Dr. von Haller was identified as cholesterol. Atherosclerosis, then, is a type of arteriosclerosis characterized by a cholesterol-laden scab that forms on the inner walls of blood vessels.

When examined under a microscope, these atheromatous plaques appear as scar tissue on the intima: each nodule contains yellowish, mushy cholesterol plus numerous white corpuscles (cells that usually seek any irritation in the body) and flecks of calcium salts that compose the plaque. Beneath the plaque, muscle fiber and elastic filaments are destroyed, resulting in the media layer being weakened and thin.

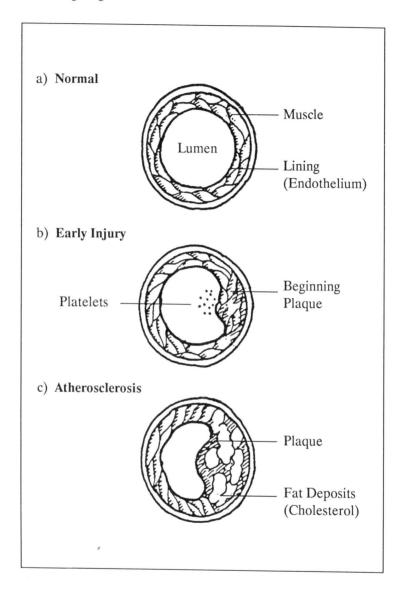

a) **Normal**

Muscle

Lumen

Lining
(Endothelium)

b) **Early Injury**

Platelets

Beginning
Plaque

c) **Atherosclerosis**

Plaque

Fat Deposits
(Cholesterol)

FIGURE 2
MAGNIFIED CROSS-SECTIONS OF BLOOD VESSELS
SHOWING ATHEROSCLEROSIS

What aggravates or accelerates the development of these plaques? Physicians believe that plaque formation commences when the delicate intima lining of an artery is damaged by the constant rough and tumble of blood passing through channels under high pressure; or it may be triggered by the effect of a high level of stress with an excess of the hormone *epinephrine*; or it may result from eating too much fat, saturated fat, and cholesterol. When serum cholesterol levels are high, the damaged area of the artery is transformed into plaque having a core of cholesterol and a cap of calcium. Over a period of ten, twenty or thirty years, a mixture of dead and dying cells, fat, clotted blood and deposits of flinty calcium can progressively encrust inner artery walls. With these thick, rough deposits of plaque, atherosclerosis narrows the channel like a kettle acquiring "fur," slows the flow of blood, and makes clot formation more likely. Blood is designed to clot when it comes in contact with foreign substances, and as plaque builds up, the blood treats the plaque as an alien substance − the result being unusual clotting referred to as embolisms which can cause a heart attack or stroke. Many people with severe atherosclerosis have no symptoms until a blood clot forms or arterial plaque builds up to completely block blood flow. You don't feel pain until it is too late and you are struck down with sudden death or paralysis.

Atherosclerosis most commonly affects the function of the heart or the brain, but it can also clog other arteries. A clot which forms in an arm or leg blood vessel can block blood flow to the limb or a clot can disconnect from its original site and be carried in the bloodstream until it stops in another part of the body. When blocked arteries provide an inadequate blood supply to extremities, the condition is known as *peripheral vascular disease* (PVD) which can then lead to gangrene (decomposition), and aneurysms (unusual dilation of the arteries) in other body tissues. Aneurysms may burst with disastrous results. Diabetics are particularly at risk of developing PVD which accounts for many amputations performed on people with diabetes.

The Heart. To keep blood moving around your circulatory system, your heart beats about 100,000 times a day, continuously pumping about 10 pints (5 liters) of blood per minute – 15,000 pints (7,000 liters) of blood every 24 hours. The amount of blood pumped by the heart decreases with age: assuming your heart is functioning at 100 percent capacity when you are thirty years of age, its efficiency is down to 80 percent by the time you are fifty and to 70 percent by the time you are eighty. The beat goes on inside each of us – unnoticed – until something goes wrong.

Clench your fist and that will give you a rough idea of the size of your heart. This muscle, weighing about 2/3 ounce (19g) in a newborn and between 9 and 12 ounces (250 and 350g) in an adult, keeps the blood circulating whether you are in deep sleep or exercising vigorously. The heart is not the frail mystical thing that we might believe it to be, but a device with immense hardiness and an amazing ability to repair itself after injury. However, like any other muscle, the heart must have a constant supply of fresh blood to keep working – blood that brings oxygen and chemical nutrients.

The heartbeat arises in the specialized muscle that comprises the bulk of the organ, the *myocardium*, which is programmed genetically to contract and relax on its own. The prompting for the beat originates with an electrical impulse from the heart's own natural pacemaker, the *sinoatrial node*, that causes the heart muscle to contract 60 to 80 times a minute – or quicker or slower according to the demands you make of it. Chemical energy received from glucose, fats and oxygen is converted into mechanical movement, these substances being carried to the heart-muscle cells by the bloodstream. All of the blood for your heart must pass through the lungs to pick up oxygen and discharge waste gases, just as food must be absorbed through the intestinal wall.

The heart is suspended between the lungs in the center of your chest. You may have thought it was on your left side, but that is because the beat from the powerful left chamber, the left *ventricle*, sounds most strongly on the left side of the chest. The left ventricle has three times as much muscle as the right as it has been given more work to do; it accepts refreshed blood from the lungs and pumps it to the rest of the body. The right ventricle accepts the carbon dioxide-laden blood returning from circulating through the body and pushes it into the lungs.

The hypothalamus region in the brain coordinates signals that make the heart respond almost instantly to external stimulants — changes in body temperature, coffee and tea, fatigue, fever, and so on — via hormonal messages in the bloodstream and nervous system.

Nearly all the parts that keep the heart functioning smoothly can be affected by disease, infection and even normal wear and tear. Thousands of babies every year are born with heart defects that can impair proper functioning. Heart valves can be damaged by rheumatic heart disease. The electrical impulse system can be damaged by bacteria or worn down sufficiently to change the rhythm, causing dizzy feelings or tiredness due to poor circulation through the heart. The arteries that serve the heart can be plugged in later years by cholesterol-laden clogs so that the muscle is starved of its blood supply, causing a heart attack.

The pulse. Your doctor will probably take your pulse rate when you visit his office. He also may advise you to take your own pulse rate regularly if you already have heart problems, wear a pacemaker, have had open-heart surgery, or are taking medicine that may affect your heart.

Checking a pulse is easy once you know where to feel for the light throb that the blood makes as the heart pumps it through your body. The best spots are at the inner wrist or at the neck (either side of your Adam's apple) where major arteries run just beneath the skin. Place your index and middle fingers lightly over the artery without too much pressure, which would obstruct the flow. Using a watch or clock that indicates seconds, count the throbs which correspond exactly to your heartbeats. Count the beats for 15 seconds and multiply the number by 4.

Normal pulse rate when resting or sitting quietly can vary widely, ranging between 60 and 80 beats per minute; healthy people can have resting pulses as low as 35 or as high as 100.

Excitement or exertion can accelerate the beat up to as much as 200 beats per minute. Your doctor can tell you if your rate is abnormal or an indication of illness.

According to researchers from the Framingham Heart Study in Massachusetts, reporting in the *American Heart Journal*, the normal rate statistically is 72 beats per minute. Although there are some minor variations by age and sex, it appears that slow heart rates of between 30 and 67 beats per minute in a healthy person are related to a significantly decreased risk of heart disease and death due to underlying heart problems. Slower heart rates are often associated with programs of regular physical exercise and the effective management of stress. The highest rates of heart disease are among people with pulse rates of 92 to 220 per minute.

The Electrocardiogram (EKG or ECG). Your physician may use a machine to capture the heart's electrical impulse as it is discharged (without interfering with any of the body's functions), and record it on paper or on a fluorescent screen. No electricity flows into your body from the equipment — the flow is going in the opposite direction, through electrodes placed on the chest and arms. The peaks and dips from this graph of voltage can help your doctor detect heart trouble by seeing any minor irregularities in the pattern. The EKG is no crystal ball, however, and cannot predict what your heart will do in the future, but the doctor can see on the EKG strip if any abnormal discharges are occurring during the test, and he can be alerted to problems.

Prothrombin time. Another test that your doctor may want to perform is a measure of prothrombin time, to see how quickly your blood clots in a test tube, normally 10.5 to 12.5 seconds. The result sometimes is given as a percentage of normal clotting time. Longer-than-normal prothrombin time can indicate that additional tests are needed for possible inherited blood disorders, liver disease, bile duct obstructions or other problems. Certain medicines can prolong or accelerate prothrombin time.

WHAT IS A HEART ATTACK?

In most cases when a heart attack occurs, fatty deposits composed mostly of cholesterol have lined the coronary arteries. Arteries are progressively narrowed as the deposits build up, until the flow of blood to the heart is decreased or stopped. Inadequate blood to the heart muscle causes chest pains known as *angina pectoris*. With a decrease in flow to the heart, the heart muscle may be damaged; with a complete blockage of blood flow, the heart is unable to receive the oxygen and nutrients it needs, resulting in part of the heart actually dying.

A heart attack usually is the result of a blood clot forming in an already-narrowed artery and blocking the flow of blood to the part of the heart muscle serviced by that artery. This form of heart attack is called a *coronary thrombosis, coronary occlusion* or *myocardial infarction*.

When a heart attack occurs, the dying part of the heart may trigger unusual electrical activity to cause blood to be pumped to the organs of the body. Quite often, if a doctor or trained professional is immediately available, the heart can be made to beat again by using electrical shock and/or drugs. Most ambulances now carry special equipment called defibrillators. Skilled First-Aiders who know cardiopulmonary resuscitation (CPR) can mean the difference between life and death; CPR involves using a combination of mouth-to-mouth resuscitation to maintain a victim's breathing, and compression of the chest to maintain circulation. A heart-attack victim may be able to remain conscious until help arrives by using a "do-it-yourself" CPR technique – coughing vigorously about once every second.

If not too much heart muscle is damaged, and if the heart can continue beating, blood may be rerouted around the blocked arteries by means of small blood vessels, which is the heart's own way of circumventing the obstruction.

Following a heart attack there may be irregular heartbeats known as *arrhythmias*, when the heart's natural pacemaker may not be working properly, causing an irregular rhythm, or a fast or slow rate.

When there has been damage to the heart muscle, the condition is called *congestive heart failure* (CHF), most commonly due to atherosclerosis or high blood pressure. The damage results in the heart muscle pumping less effectively, circulation being inadequate, with subsequent congestion in tissues.

The most common time for a fatal heart attack appears to be immediately after rising in the morning, when the body is gearing up for the day's later demands; blood pressure is rising, heart rate is increasing and platelets are becoming more prone to cause a blood clot.

How will you know if you are having a heart attack?

Although not all symptoms necessarily occur, most usual is a feeling of uncomfortable pressure, squeezing or pain in the center of your chest, possibly spreading to your shoulders, neck or arms. You may also sweat, feel dizzy and faint, have a feeling of acute indigestion or sickness, or have shortness of breath. On the other hand, sharp, stabbing twinges are *not* usually signals of a heart attack. But the key to survival is recognizing the warning signals, and getting immediate medical attention.

Angiography. The best way for your doctor to diagnose angina is for you to undergo cardiac angiography, where X-rays are taken of your heart after an opaque dye has been injected into the coronary arteries. This gives a clear picture of the heart's blood supply.

WHAT IS A STROKE?

A stroke (or apoplexy) occurs when an area of brain tissue dies because its blood supply has been cut off or decreased. As with other tissues, your brain cells must have a continuous, sufficient supply of oxygen-rich blood in order to function. The brain demands 25 percent of the body's oxygen supply and receives 15 percent of the blood pumped by the heart through the carotid arteries. A stroke occurs when this flow to the brain is blocked. Brain cells can live only for a few minutes if blood supply stops (as when the heart stops beating in cardiac arrest), and cells die when denied oxygen and nutrients. Strokes from such blockages are called *ischemic strokes* or *infarctions* (just as death of part of the heart muscle is called a myocardial infarction).

There are three major types of stroke: *thrombotic, embolic* and *hemorrhagic.* The blockages are caused by a clot — a thrombus or embolus, depending on where the clot formed. The most common type, thrombotic, arises when arteries in the head or neck become partly clogged by fatty deposits of atherosclerosis. Blood flow around obstructions is slowed, so clots can form and lodge in the clogged vessel. When this occurs, it is referred to as a *cerebral thrombosis.* The peak age for this type of stroke is seventy years. An embolic stroke occurs when a wandering blood clot from a diseased artery in another part of the body (most often the heart or lungs) lodges in one of the cerebral arteries, causing obstruction and choking off the flow of blood; this stroke is called a *cerebral embolism.* A stroke also happens when a damaged artery bursts in the brain, flooding the surrounding tissue with blood. This is referred to as a *cerebral hemorrhage.* About 15 percent of all strokes are hemorrhagic and are fatal in about 50 percent of cases. Cerebral hemorrhage is more likely to occur if you suffer from a combination of hardening of the arteries (atherosclerosis) and uncontrolled high blood pressure.

As brain cells die, the functions they control die with them or are impaired. A stroke usually paralyzes one side of the body, with loss of speech or an understanding of others' speech, and possibly loss of memory. Brain cells injured by a stroke cannot heal or create new cells, and the effects may be slight or severe, temporary or permanent, depending on the extent of the damage, which cells have been affected, and how well the body restores its blood supply.

How will you know if you are suffering a stroke?
About 10 percent of the time, there is advance warning of a coming stroke in the form of one or more *transient ischemic attacks* (TIAs). A TIA is a kind of mini-stroke which signals that the flow of blood to the brain has been temporarily interrupted,

in most cases by tiny clots (emboli) that have broken loose from plaque in heart or neck arteries. Depending on the part of the brain affected, a TIA can cause a sudden weakness or numbness of the face, arm or leg on one side of the body. Other symptoms include temporary difficulty in speaking or writing, blindness (particularly in one eye), sudden falls, puzzling dizziness or unsteadiness. The attack usually lasts less than thirty minutes – hence the term transient, but it is important to report it to your doctor as a TIA is a strong predictor of stroke. About 30 percent of people who have had one, can expect a stroke within five years. Your doctor can determine whether the problem is caused by atherosclerosis.

Peripheral vascular disease. If you are over the age of fifty, watch for these warning signals of an inadequate supply of blood to lower limbs:

  a) aching, cramping or pain in the legs when you walk or
    exercise, which disappears after rest.
  b) occasional tingling, numbness or coldness in hands or feet.
  c) loss of hair on feet or toes.
  d) irregularity in the growth of fingernails or toenails.

WHAT ARE YOUR CHANCES OF SUFFERING CARDIOVASCULAR DISEASE?

Many factors contribute to the development of vascular diseases. Some of these factors are controllable; others are totally beyond your influence. After a heart attack, many patients modify their behavior pattern in an attempt to improve or eliminate abnormal risk factors. Isn't it absurd to wait to change your ways of living until *after* a heart attack? Why not change your lifestyle *now* and perhaps avoid an attack?

You cannot change:
  - Your sex
  - Race
  - Age
  - Heredity
  - Previous disease

But you can control:
- Eating properly
- Drinking in moderation
- Checking blood pressure
- Checking cholesterol
- Stopping smoking, or not starting

- Watching your weight
- Diabetes
- Trying to relax and enjoy life
- Drug abuse
- Taking more exercise

Sex. You cannot change your sex hormones. The male hormone testosterone causes men to have a far higher concentration of LDLs which attach to the linings of blood vessels making them narrower and more fragile. On the other hand, estrogens in women keep the blood vessels pliable (so that they may accommodate extra blood volume during pregnancy) thus reducing the risk of atherosclerosis in women. In addition, estrogen stimulates the liver to produce HDLs to help keep arteries cleared of cholesterol. Young women seem to have the advantage of a much lower death rate from heart attack than men, but women smokers cancel out some of that advantage. When women undergo hysterectomy and removal of both ovaries, surgical menopause causes the abrupt cessation of natural estrogen, more than doubling the risk of coronary disease unless they receive replacement estrogen. With estrogen therapy, they are at no more risk than premenopausal women of the same age. Women who use estrogen supplements after menopause cut their risk of heart attacks by a third.

Race. In the U.S., black Americans are nearly 44 percent more likely to have heart disease, because their incidence of high blood pressure is twice that of whites. According to statistics, they are also more likely to suffer strokes at an earlier age and with greater severity. However in Britain, a study of black and white workers in Birmingham showed that blood pressure on average is no different in blacks in Britain (first generation immigrants from the West Indies) than in whites.

Age. Almost a quarter of all heart attack deaths occur before the age of 65. Stroke, usually considered a disease of the elderly, also strikes younger people. One in seven people who die from stroke are under the age of 65.

Heredity. Family history is a powerful predictor. So it's important to know the medical history of your parents, grandparents, brothers and sisters. Some families have inherited susceptibility to heart disease. You may have inherited the problem of your body naturally manufacturing too much cholesterol, or you may not be able to eliminate the cholesterol that you consume. More than 1 million people lack the ability to remove LDL from their blood and as a result have very high LDL cholesterol levels by age one or two, a condition known as *familial hypercholesterolemia*. Their average age for heart attack is 45. About 2 million people have inherited *familial combined hyperlipidemia*, with higher LDL levels, high triglycerides, or a combination. Disorders start in the teen years and the average age for heart attack is 55. Yet another segment of the population has inherited normally low levels of the protective HDL cholesterol, giving an increased risk of heart attack even if total cholesterol is not high.

If you belong to a high-risk family, it could be a matter of life and death to know CPR techniques in an emergency, before the arrival of paramedics or the doctor. Enrol at least one family member in a First Aid course to learn the correct methods. Phone your local chapter of the American Heart Association or the American Red Cross for information.

Previous disease. You may have had heart irregularities from birth, had heart valves damaged from rheumatic heart disease, or had previous heart surgery that may make you more vulnerable in later years to unusual blood clotting.

WHAT YOU CAN CONTROL
Even if you fall into any of the higher risk groups, you may still minimize your risk by –

Eating properly. Have a well-balanced diet to meet your daily need for protein, vitamins, minerals and other nutrients. The way to a man's heart is still through his stomach, but the old saying has taken on a second meaning: the food you eat can endanger your heart – or protect it, with a reduction in the total amount of fat, especially saturates and cholesterol. Limit fat to no more than 30 percent and saturates to 10 percent. It is also a good idea to keep your intake of sugar low and cut back on the coffee and tea you drink. There is a theory that diets high in sugar are an important cause of atherosclerosis and heart disease, but there is a much stronger correlation world wide between fat consumption and cardiovascular disease.

Drinking in moderation. The odds of getting vascular diseases are increased if you drink heavily. If you drink alcohol, do so in moderation. Actually, moderate amounts may fractionally elevate HDL that is not protective against heart disease.

Checking your blood pressure. According to *The Surgeon-General's Report on Nutrition and Health*, 1988, 58 million Americans suffer from high blood pressure. In many cases of hypertension, the cause is unknown, but the effects are well known. High blood pressure damages arteries and weakens your heart by overloading it. Your heart is forced to pump harder than normal, causing it to enlarge and weaken, resulting in potential heart failure. With high blood pressure (160/95 or greater), strokes occur two to four times more frequently. About 95 percent of people with hypertension have it because of extra weight from overeating, chronic stress, or the loss of the kidneys' ability to handle salt. During pregnancy, hypertension can develop very rapidly, which is why physicians and clinical workers measure blood pressure frequently. Hypertension can also occur in children, although cases are generally mild and usually found in families with histories of high blood pressure and excess body weight. Hypertension can often be controlled by losing weight, restriction of fats and salt, a reduction in alcohol, stopping smoking and taking more exercise. Chicago researchers reported in the Spring of 1987 that a maintained weight loss of only 10 pounds, or cutting daily intake of table salt by one-third, or cutting alcohol intake in half, restored 40 percent of mild-to-moderate hypertensive patients to normal. Table salt is a villain. An important part of controlling blood pressure is a reduction in the amount of salt and sodium you eat. As an adult, your body needs little more than 200mg of sodium each day – the amount in only 1/10 of a teaspoon of salt. Generally, you should have no more than 1000mg of sodium for every 1000 calories you consume. Saccharin, a common sweetener, contains no calories but considerable sodium. Put away your saltshaker, and add zest to food flavors with fresh herbs [See *THE SODIUM-WATCHER'S GUIDE: Easy Ways to Cut Salt and Sodium*, Pennant Books]. Several investigations over the years have found that a high intake of potassium (found in generous amounts of fruits and vegetables) can protect against hypertension.

Your doctor can prescribe antihypertensive drugs, although these may produce side effects of weakness, fatigue, dizziness, impotence and allergies. For this reason, alternative non-drug lifestyle changes are often sufficient and preferable.

Checking your cholesterol. More than 60 million Americans may have blood cholesterol levels that are too high. Do you know *your* current level? Cholesterol is now considered one of the major health barometers. It is the cholesterol in your bloodstream that is measured for cholesterol readings: the simple procedure involves your doctor taking a few drops of blood from a pricked finger for laboratory analysis, and it should be a regular practice when you are examined by your physician or health professional. In the U.S., cholesterol-testing devices calibrated to the Abell-Kendall reference method are generally used. Sometimes the doctor will ask the laboratory to report LDL and HDL as well as blood cholesterol, and with these tests for triglycerides you usually have to fast for several hours beforehand. Your physician can tell you what steps are necessary if your cholesterol is too high for a healthy heart. More important than total blood cholesterol is the amount of protective HDL cholesterol relative to the artery-damaging LDL cholesterol. An increase in LDL and a decrease in HDL levels may indicate that fat is being deposited in the linings of blood vessels, or you may have inherited hypercholesterolemia, high serum cholesterol not connected with the amount of cholesterol you eat. While you cannot directly eat HDL cholesterol, various foods can help increase the relative amount circulating in your blood.

Blood cholesterol levels are measured in milligrams per deciliter of blood. Levels tend to rise with age, probably because of the tendency to eat greater amounts of saturated fats. The average middle-aged American now has a cholesterol level of 215 milligrams (mg)/deciliter (dl). You may have had your cholesterol measured at one time and been told only that it was "normal." But standards have changed, and what was once considered normal is now widely thought to be too high. It's best to have it checked every five years.

In October 1987, a federal advisory panel convened by the National Heart, Lung and Blood Institute, set simplified practical guidelines for physicians when measuring blood cholesterol in everyone aged 20 or older:

Total cholesterol:	Category:
Below 200mg/dl	Desirable blood cholesterol
200 to 239mg/dl	Borderline high cholesterol
240mg/dl or above	High blood cholesterol

Generally speaking, any count below 200mg/dl is considered safe, but the lower the better. Since many people with levels between 150 and 200 suffer heart attacks, an ideal cholesterol level is really under 150. If you are over 40 years of age, with blood cholesterol above 260, you are at high risk and should be treated. The National Heart, Lung and Blood Institute states that people with blood cholesterol over 260 have four times the risk of developing heart disease compared to those with a level of 190 or lower. High blood cholesterol may also trigger the formation of gallstones in the gallbladder.

If you are classified as having "borderline high cholesterol" you may be given dietary information and retested 6 months or a year later. If you have a cholesterol level of 240 or higher, specific LDL cholesterol analysis may be called for, classified as follows:

LDL cholesterol:	Category:
130 to 159mg/dl	Borderline high-risk LDL
160 mg/dl or above	High-risk LDL

About 30 percent of youngsters in the U.S. are estimated to have abnormally high blood cholesterol levels. By age four, the average American child has already reached a level of serum cholesterol as high as it should be in adulthood if coronary arteries are to remain unclogged by fatty acids. Throughout the world, cholesterol levels of children closely correlate to those of adults (with the exception of Japan, where adults have long had very low levels of cholesterol and low incidence of heart disease. Today's children, however, have disproportionately high levels of cholesterol suggesting a steady increase in heart disease will occur as they age).

Cholesterol and triglyceride levels can sometimes be controlled by drugs such as cholestyramine, colestipol, lovastatin or niacin. Niacin (or nicotinic acid) is available from pharmacies without a doctor's prescription. Some of these drugs can create problems: Lovastatin may promote eye cataracts; others can cause possible depletion of vitamins, a change in liver function, headaches, constipation, feeling bloated and flushed, activation of peptic ulcers, and in some cases gouty arthritis. The American Medical Association recommends that a change in diet is often more effective, generally safer, and should be tried first.

Americans now consume between 350mg and 450mg of cholesterol daily — down from 700mg of a few years ago. But experts recommend a limit of 100mg per 1,000 calories, and no more than 300mg per day, plus an increase in fiber intake to more than 30g per day.

If you have an average diet, most of your blood cholesterol originates with the cholesterol and saturated fats you eat: eggs, meats, processed luncheon meats and organ meats (liver, kidneys, heart, brains, sweetbreads, paté) and whole-milk dairy products. One large whole egg has over 200mg of cholesterol, concentrated in the yolk. Your local supermarket may be selling reduced-cholesterol eggs, but these may still have more cholesterol than you want. These are the food items you should be cutting back while substituting fish, PUFAs and soluble fibers as in oats, apples, dried beans and peas. There can be some tradeoffs involved in heart-healthy eating: liver, for example, is high in cholesterol (about 440mg per 3 1/2 oz portion) but the American Heart Association recommends eating it at least once a month for its high levels of other beneficial nutrients.

The next question is: what about your children? Should their diet be altered? Although the slow, symptomless buildup of cholesterol in arteries can begin early in life, pediatricians recommend that the problem should only be considered after the age of two years. The American Academy of Pediatrics recommends breast milk for the first four to six months of life. Breast milk, Nature's ideal food for babies, contains between 40 percent and 50 percent of its calories from fat, about half saturated and half unsaturated, and about 150mg of cholesterol per deciliter (about one-tenth of a quart). When you start giving cows' milk to infants, the Academy suggests that it be whole (not lowfat or skim). Although the American Academy of Pediatrics does not recommend cholesterol screening for all children, it does suggest monitoring every child older than two where there is a family history of cardiovascular disease. Your doctor or clinic will take into consideration whether close relatives have suffered premature heart attack or stroke, hypertension, obesity, diabetes and the various types of inherited hyperlipidemias or hypercholesterolemia.

Because eggs and organ meats are the primary sources of cholesterol in our food supply, nutritionists consider that they should be restricted for teenage boys, when hormonal changes that seem related to cholesterol buildup in young men begin to take place. Carefully check their consumption of saturates, cholesterol and salt, and substitute PUFA oils. For total fat intake, 30 to 40 percent of calories from fat appears to be sensible for adequate growth and development – similar to the recommended prudent guidelines for adults, but with a little more leeway.

Stopping smoking, or not starting. Don't smoke cigarettes! The link between smoking and heart attack and other heart diseases is established beyond a doubt. Nicotine in smoke makes the heart beat faster and stronger, and boosts blood pressure, while inhaled smoke constricts blood vessels. When carbon monoxide from smoke is in the lungs, it decreases the amount of oxygen carried by red blood cells and thus deprives the heart of oxygen. In addition, a tobacco substance called *rutin* appears to promote clot formation. Cigarette smokers have twice the risk of heart attack as nonsmokers; up to four times the risk of sudden cardiac death. Autopsies of smokers show that their arteries are generally harder and thicker due to atherosclerosis than those of nonsmokers. If you have been smoking for twenty years and you stop right now, you can still dramatically reduce your risk. The fewer cigarettes you smoke, the lower your risk of heart disease.

Watching your weight. Obesity results in an additional strain on your heart. Weight loss can reduce blood pressure and serum cholesterol levels, and the risk of developing diabetes. Research studies have noted that the heart seems immediately relieved when weight declines and it no longer has to pump blood to excess fatty tissues. See Chapter 5 "Fats and Weight Control."

Watching out for diabetes. Diabetes, or an inherited tendency towards it, is linked with an increased risk of heart attack and stroke, because of abnormal metabolism of fats as well as sugars. You are more liable to suffer Type II diabetes if overweight and middle-aged. Mild forms of diabetes can remain undetected for years. Because diabetes sharply increases your risk of heart attack, controlling the other risk factors − such as blood pressure, blood fats and cholesterol − is even more important. Glucose is the sugar the body forms from dietary starches and other carbohydrates and, in small amounts, from fat metabolism. Normal levels, measured after overnight fasting, range between 70 and 110mg per deciliter of blood. Higher levels of blood glucose might indicate diabetes. Your doctor can detect diabetes and prescribe a special program of diet, weight control, exercise, and medicines if appropriate. Home test-kits allow diabetics to monitor blood-sugar levels constantly, and to alter insulin use or diet as necessary.

Recent studies in the U.S. and Britain have shown that a near-vegetarian diet, high in fiber and complex carbohydrates, is ideal for control of Type II diabetes, with fats only 10 percent of calories. Diabetics under the guidance of a physician can vastly improve their control of blood sugar by reducing dietary fat as well as their sugar intake.

Trying to relax and enjoy life. Stress is with us most of the time. Stress can put a strain on your life. What may be stimulating to one person may be stressful to another. We're all different. Stress comes from emotional activity and from physical activity. But while physical activity can help you relax, too much emotional stress can cause distress and physical illness. It can have a positive influence, but here it means a negative force. The body reacts to unusual stress with a complicated "fight-flight" syndrome, pumping adrenalin and speeding up the heart, sending more blood to the brain and muscles. Blood pressure rises to dangerous levels; the liver dumps cholesterol into the bloodstream.

Some researchers believe that sex hormones dictate the difference in the way men and women react to stress. Testosterone can be blamed for men's response to stress in two ways: one mechanical and the other chemical. Mechanically, it elevates the heart rate and blood pressure, thus promoting damage to the inner lining of arteries. And chemically, testosterone orders neuroreceptors in the brain to react to the release of stress hormones, and this increased production of stress hormones promotes arterial damage. On the other hand, women seem to respond to stressful situations more slowly, with less of a surge of blood pressure and stress hormones. Estrogens may be better adapted than testosterone for the fight-flight situations in modern life.

Stress can be from internal turmoil, if you are worrying over a personal illness or injury; or you may be feeling frayed by external factors: the death of a close relative, family problems, money problems, noisy neighbors, unbearable workloads or overtime, chronic frustration with tyrannical supervisors, unemployment, retirement, driving in rush-hour traffic. Anxiety, boredom and grief.

How do you cope? There is no single strategy that is best for everyone. You can face up to the problems and take direct action to solve them. Or rationalize the situation and avoid dealing with painful issues. Or accept the problem("I can't do anything about it anyway") and make no attempt to change anything. Look on the bright side. Ways to relax can include −

1. exercising. Do something energetic instead of giving way to anger or bottling it up: take a walk, play a friendly game of tennis, or do gardening. Deep breathing helps to relieve tension,

2. taking time to relax. Take short naps, try meditation, seek out the beauty around you, read a book, do a jigsaw puzzle, listen to beautiful music, resolve to take more vacations,

3. developing new interests, new hobbies, to help you forget daily problems: fly a kite, play a musical instrument, or go fishing. Have a pet you can play with and love,

4. seeking advice, forgiveness or an apology. Try cooperation instead of confrontation. Discuss problems with a friend you can trust, a counselor or your clergyman,

5. having a good cry now and then, as a healthy way to relieve anxiety,

6. knowing your limits. Take a slower approach to life if you are struggling to fit too many activities into your day, with family responsibilities, work, church and school.

Realize that you cannot be so ambitious. Change jobs,
maybe. List priorities – do one thing at a time and
postpone the rest,

7. getting enough rest and eating sensibly. If you are
irritable and tense from lack of sleep, or if you are not
eating right, you will be less able to deal with stressful
situations. If stress repeatedly prevents you from sleeping,
ask your doctor for help.

Drug Abuse. To relieve anxieties, be sure you are not substituting negative ways instead of positive methods. Tranquilizers, sleeping pills and other crutches may create more stress
than they take away. Take them only on your doctor's advice.

Stroke can be caused by amphetamines, cocaine and "Ts and
Blues" (pentazocine and tripelennamine). Heroin and LSD also
lead to stroke. Break the habit of drug dependence. Find out
what programs are available to you for help with drug abuse,
either through your physician, health clinic or local authorities.

Taking more regular exercise. Regular exercise conditions the
heart and most of the rest of your body, by enlarging the
diameter of the main coronary arteries and increasing the
number of blood vessels that serve the heart muscle. Exercise
brings a greater efficiency of the oxygen supply to muscles, and
can help counter diabetes with better use of the insulin
produced by the body. Exercise helps to lower blood pressure,
alter LDL and HDL levels to favorable ratios, increasing the
amount of protective HDLs and lowering the artery-damaging
LDLs, reduce blood triglyceride levels and maintain proper
weight. Researchers have found that trained athletes have a
lower level of stress hormones in their blood and a higher level
of natural tranquilizing hormones.

But you don't have to train for the Olympics or run a mara-
thon every day to gain benefits. Just bear in mind that *every* body
needs exercise, and that exercise in one form or another can be
found to suit everyone – any kind is better than none. Just a
couple of 15-minute brisk walks every day are helpful. A walk

that doesn't even cause you to break into a sweat can improve your fitness. Light gardening (rhythmic raking of leaves, sweeping paths or pushing a lawn mower) can be a significant aerobic activity to have you drinking in oxygen – not gasping for air and stopping after a burst of effort. "Aerobic" is one of those words that fitness people like to use, but it means any exercise that stimulates heart and lung activity with fresh supplies of oxygen, for a period long enough to produce beneficial changes in your body – and benefits are what fitness is all about.

Appendix II provides a list of various activities and exercises. Note that not all activities have conditioning value; some promote muscular strength, while others are better for cardiovascular fitness if you perform them briskly and continuously for a certain length of time.

Although, in general, exercise is good for most people, if you have high blood pressure, weight training can be dangerous. When you lift weights or use strength-training machines, your muscles contract against resistance. If you hold your breath, with pressure on your lungs, your heart must beat harder to pump blood, causing blood pressure to rise. And while stretching done in yoga can reduce stress and produce a sense of tranquillity, this form of exercise has no benefit in improving the function of the heart.

The effort of aerobic exercise that aims to drive your heart close to its maximum capacity for 20 or 30 minutes several times a week can make a healthy heart more efficient – but it may damage one that is not so healthy. There may be some danger if you have been sedentary and suddenly take up strenuous exercise, so it's essential to consult your doctor before commencing a regular exercise program, especially if you're over 40. But careful medical preparation is only necessary for aerobic exercise, and you can judge your own capacity for activities that are less arduous. The key to enjoying exercise is to find out how much you need to feel good, and not do more until you feel ready for it.

Walking, bicycling and swimming are good for cardiovascular conditioning because they can be continuous, keep your heart rate up, burn up calories and are more easily measured.

Walking can improve circulation, lower blood pressure, tone up your muscles, act as a natural tranquilizer, and be a tonic to your digestive system. Major health benefits can come from five 30-minute purposeful walks a week. Some people strap on 5 or 10 pound ankle- or wrist-weights, but you can get more out of walking just by holding a child or bags of groceries. The point is to walk as briskly as possible to get your heart going and activate your calorie-burning mechanism.

Bicycling can easily be a part of your regular exercise, paced according to your ability, and giving a good cardiovascular workout. You probably already have a bike in the garage or garden shed just waiting for you to brush off the cobwebs. To avoid any risk from riding on the open road, stationary bicycling provides the same benefits in the comfort of your home or garden. No weather to contend with, no highway dangers, and no dogs to attack you. You can either get a stand to modify a standard bicycle for use indoors, or buy an exercycle with the extra advantage of an adjustable resistance mechanism giving you the same workout as riding a bike uphill. To get the most out of bicycling, you should cycle a minimum of 20 minutes at least three times a week.

Swimming can be for the out-of-shape, the elderly, the obese and the arthritic. Cardiovascular activity in water can be a better, harder workout than any on land. Pushing and pulling against water adds great resistance, but because your body is supported there is almost no risk of injury, especially to the joints. Your effective body weight is less, but the water provides resistance that intensifies each movement without unnecessary stress. Try to swim three times a week, using a variety of strokes.

If you are really serious about exercising, to get the most out of it for heart strengthening, you need to pace yourself properly by measuring your pulse and knowing your "target zone." You will want to take two measurements of your pulse: one at rest and one when pacing exercise. When at rest, count the beats for 60 seconds; during exercise, count beats for 10 seconds then multiply the count by six.

Your target zone is like a speedometer; you have to look at how hard you are working to know if you have done enough. As a rule of thumb to find your target zone, subtract your age from 220. The figure that remains is your *maximum* heart rate. The exercise level you are aiming at is *60 to 75 percent* of your maximum heart rate, for example:

Age	Target Zone	Age	Target Zone
20	120 - 150	50	102 - 127
25	117 - 146	55	99 - 123
30	114 - 142	60	96 - 120
35	111 - 138	65	93 - 116
40	108 - 135	70	90 - 112
45	105 - 131	75	87 - 109

(Source: *Exercise and Your Heart*, U.S. National Heart, Lung and Blood Institute)

Exercise can help you in your fight against cardiovascular disease, but it cannot negate the damage done by a cholesterol-raising diet — you need to combine it with eating balanced meals and reduced amounts of fat. If you think you can get away with a steady diet of burgers, French fries and shakes because you run or jog every day, you're deluding yourself.

Now look at Table 4 which summarizes the major risk factors in cardiovascular disease. Sharpen your pencil to make an assessment of your own vulnerability. The test will only give you a general idea of where you stand and is not meant to replace tests performed by your doctor. The quiz provides the average risk for the average person.

MEDICATIONS THAT CAN BE HARMFUL

Discuss with your doctor any medications or supplements that you are presently taking.

Anabolic steroids, for instance, can trigger a heart attack by raising blood levels of LDL cholesterol and lowering HDL cholesterol. They are sometimes prescribed to promote weight gain

TABLE 4
RISK CHART FOR CARDIOVASCULAR DISEASE

Factors	Low	Moderate	High	Your risk
		Risk level		
Age	0 to 29	30 to 49	50 and over	_____
Family history of heart disease	None	Developed after the age of 50	Developed before the age of 50	_____
Body weight	Near optimum	10% to 20% overweight	20% or more overweight	_____
Smoking	None	Up to 10 cigarettes per day	10 or more cigarettes per day	_____
Stress	Easy going	Sometimes anxious	Always anxious and nervous	_____
Blood pressure: Systolic Diastolic	Less than 140 Less than 85	140 to 159 85 to 114	160 or more 115 or more	_____ _____
Blood cholesterol	Below 200	200 to 239	Over 240	_____
Usual food pattern	Nearly vegetarian, rare egg, lowfat dairy products	Mostly lean meat, some eggs, lowfat dairy products	Big portions of meat, fast foods, whole eggs, whole dairy products	_____
Exercise	Vigorous and regular	Occasionally	Rarely	_____
Drinking alcohol	None	One glass per day	More than one glass per day	_____
Diabetes	None	Mild	Insulin dependent	_____

in underweight people, or are given to athletes to build muscle mass. In Finland, a study group of people over the age of 60 were given anabolic steroids to strengthen their bones. But this experiment was stopped because a high percentage of these people taking steroids suffered heart attacks. In young people whose arteries are relatively free from plaques, the impact of steroids may not occur immediately, because it takes years for plaques to build in the arteries. However, the arteries of most older people already contain a lot of plaques, so it would not take much more to close arteries and cause a heart attack.

Steroid or **cortisone drugs** for asthmatics can raise blood pressure.

Cold and **allergy preparations** may stimulate your heart and raise blood pressure. People who already have high blood pressure may be sensitive to oral decongestants.

Some **appetite-suppressant drugs** used in the management of weight control, such as diethylpropion, mazindol and phentermine, can produce *tachycardia* (a heartbeat rate that is abnormally fast when you are at rest) so these drugs are unsuitable if you have angina.

Over-supplementation of **calcium tablets** may trigger a buildup of calcium along artery walls and aggravate arteriosclerosis, but at the same time calcium supplements have a mild blood pressure lowering effect.

Blood pressure may rise if you are prescribed **estrogen**, due to the action of two enzymes, renin and angiotensin; high-estrogen birth-control pills (more than 50 micrograms of estrogen) have been linked with blood-clotting disorders. However, estrogen therapy is also thought to promote the general health and elasticity of arteries.

MEDICATIONS THAT CAN HELP

When arteries are already seriously narrowed, blocked or clotted, your doctor may prescribe one or more of these drugs —

Heart strengtheners. Digoxin and digitoxin (derived from the foxglove plant) and others like it, strengthen the contraction of the heart muscle fibers, creating more powerful and more efficient pumping. Relatively new medications to improve the action of the heart muscle are amerinone, milrinone and enoximone.

Heartbeat regulators. Disopyramide, quinidine, procainamide and propranolol and similar drugs control heart rhythm by stabilizing electrical impulses.

Pain relievers. Beta-blockers or vasodilators. Both relieve angina. A common beta-blocker is propranolol, lowering the oxygen needs of the heart and reducing the force of contractions. In the vasodilator class of drugs, such as prazosin and hydralazine and nitroglycerin, blood vessels are dilated, lowering blood pressure.

Preventives. Blood pressure can be brought down by diuretics, beta-blockers or vasodilators. Diuretics for the release of water and salt may be drugs such as hydrochlorothiazide or metolazone; beta-blockers may be propranolol; vasodilators may be hydralazine, nitroglycerin preparations, prazosin and captopril.

Anticoagulants. Low-dose aspirin is often prescribed to reduce abnormal tendencies to clotting, or the drug coumadin. One of the new drugs produced through genetic engineering techniques is tissue plasminogen factor or TPA, a human protein that disintegrates blood clots when injected into the bloodstream, thus controlling the severity of a heart attack.

Tranquilizers. To relieve chronic conditions of stress and anxiety, drugs such as diazepam and chlordiazepoxide may be prescribed.

Many drugs in these categories have to be taken for a number of years and maybe for the rest of your life. Some medicines have unpleasant side effects, but it is important to follow your physician's instructions — if you stop taking them, or take them incorrectly, it could prove fatal. Discuss with your doctor any alternatives to drug-based treatment; he may consider it possible to control certain problems with a low-fat diet, sensible daily exercise and stress management.

A DIFFERENT GRADE OF OIL

Like a quality car, your body may perform better on a different grade of oil. In this connection, researchers are investigating new classifications of dietary fatty acids called the *omega-3 polyunsaturates* that appear to inhibit the process of atherosclerosis. Chemically, omega-3 fatty acids (sometimes written as w3 or n-3) look remarkably like any other polyunsaturated fat. They differ only in the location of the double carbon bonds on the carbon chain: an omega-3 has its first double bond starting on the third carbon atom of the chain, which affects the reaction with other substances in your body.

What can omega-3s do? Omega-3 polyunsaturates, notably eicosapentaenoic acid (EPA) (20:5, omega-3) and docosahexaenoic acid (DHA) (22:6, omega-3), are metabolized in the body to compounds that –

* reduce blood pressure,
* lower total levels of cholesterol,
* change the critical balance of lipoproteins, reducing the levels of the evil LDLs and VLDLs that deposit cholesterol on artery walls, and improving their clearance from blood and excretion from the body,
* lower levels of triglycerides in people who have inherited a tendency to accumulate this form of fat,
* inhibit the formation of life-threatening blood clots by making platelets (the cells involved in clotting) less "sticky", preventing the clumping or clotting that can lead to heart attack and stroke,
* make red blood cells less rigid and more flexible, so the cells glide smoothly along the bloodstream,
* discourage arteries to close again following heart surgery.

Where can they be found? Researchers observed that Greenland Eskimos and Japanese fishermen have a much lower incidence of heart disease, though a greater incidence of stroke. Their blood cholesterol and triglyceride levels are fairly low despite a diet that tends to be high in cholesterol and fat. The difference apparently is the type of fat — the omega-3s— in the fish and whale blubber diet eaten by these people in sufficient amounts so as to alter their body chemistry, and give them benefit from its anti-inflammatory and fluid-inducing effects. Actually the source of omega-3 oil is *not* fish but microscopic organisms, the plankton on which the fish have been feeding.

Fish such as salmon, mackerel, tuna, sardines, sablefish and herring, that swim in cold ocean waters, are high in omega-3s which keep the systems of cold-water fish fluid. Omega-3s are even found in leaner fish such as cod, flounder and haddock, but in smaller quantities. Cod store most of their oil in their livers.

Exact omega-3 values are difficult to list because the lipid content of even the same fish is extremely variable according to species, sex, maturity, food supply, season, salinity and temperature of the water. The muscle fat content of herring, for example, has been found to vary anywhere from 8 percent to 40 percent. Freshwater fish from cold water, such as rainbow trout, are also good sources, but as a general rule, saltwater fish are richer in omega-3s than freshwater fish, and the colder the water, the more omega-3s.

Shellfish also contain these PUFAs, so this type of seafood can be eaten occasionally. People with high serum cholesterol had been advised for years to limit consumption of shellfish because it was generally believed to be high in cholesterol, but it turns out that this is not so, according to new research findings by the Cornell University Cooperative Extension. Past methods of measuring fats in mollusks (oysters, scallops, shrimp and crab, mussels and clams) had overestimated the amounts of cholesterol because similar chemicals — other harmless sterols — had been included.

High-fish diets are not entirely without risk. Fish is not yet subject to the same stringent systematic inspections as livestock and poultry, and fish-borne diseases such as gastroenteritis, hepatitis A and cholera appear to be on the increase around the U.S. So it is important to purchase fish and shellfish from reputable markets and to know if supplies have been harvested from safe waters. Eating deepwater ocean fish is usually safe, but fish caught in coastal waters may contain such pollutants as lead, polychlorinated biphenyls (PCBs), or other industrial chemicals from rivers and drainage ditches which can unfortunately accumulate in fatty fish. Pollution can be spread by tides, currents, wave action and storms. The toxins are likely to cause increased cancer risks, damage to the nervous system and interfere with fetal development during pregnancy. Shellfish may be exposed to naturally occurring environmental contaminants, "red tides," sewage and boat fuel. Rainbow trout raised commercially or caught from pollutant-free clear mountain streams are generally wholesome.

Concentrated fish-oil supplements can pose hazards similar to fresh fish. Health-food shops and drug stores have many fish-oil preparations usually in the form of concentrated capsules or emulsions, many of which are produced from menhaden. Since most chemical residues concentrate in the fish liver and fatty tissues, it is possible that fish-oil preparations derived from fish livers and parts of fish you don't normally eat, may be contaminated with pesticides or other potentially dangerous compounds. Cod-liver oil has been a dietary supplement for a great number of years. In Iceland, where more than a third of the world's supply is produced, the people enthusiastically consume more cod-liver oil than any other nation, believing that it contributes to healthy arteries and longevity.

Fish oils also appear useful in the treating of other diseases, relieving inflammation in arthritis and nephritis (inflammation of the kidneys) improving the insulin levels in the blood of diabetics, and easing allergies, asthma, hay fever and migraine headaches. These uses are still under investigation.

But excesses can be hazardous: cod-liver oil is high in vitamins A and D which can be toxic to the body if taken in large quantities. It is not a good idea to take cod-liver oil in amounts greater than one or two tablespoons a day in order to get EPA (some firms now market fish-oil concentrate with low levels of vitamins A and D).

Calories count too. Fish oils contain as many calories as other oils and you may have an unwelcome weight gain if you take large supplementary amounts. Doses sufficient to be of thera-peutic value may give you up to 300 extra calories a day.

If you have digestive problems, these supplements may increase your tendency to belching, and give you fish-tasting reflux.

Many doctors believe it is premature to endorse the consumption of fish-oil supplements until more is known about the benefits. There is some concern that problems may arise when people on low-cholesterol diets begin to supplement their food with fish oils because of the cholesterol content. Studies have shown that in some cases fish-oil supplements have actually worsened conditions in people who already have a blood-lipid disorder. Large amounts may be hazardous if taken with aspirin, which also inhibits blood clotting. It is unwise to self-medicate. Instead, doctors prefer to make the recommendation that rather than capsules or supplements you should get your omega-3s the way the Eskimos get theirs: eat various kinds of fish at least twice a week, instead of red meat, prepared in ways that don't use much fat. Fish should not be added to a vegetarian diet, however, as it would tend to raise serum cholesterol.

But what if you are a vegetarian, cannot eat fish or do not care to? Biochemists have been researching alternative food sources of omega-3s such as the 18:3 omega-3 in rapeseed oil, soybean lecithin, soybeans and tofu, dry beans, seaweeds, walnut oil, walnuts and wheat-germ oil. Rapeseed oil (sometimes marketed as canola oil) has been processed and used for years by Europeans, but it is still comparatively new to Americans and is starting to be blended into cooking oils. Purslane (*portulaca oleracea sativa*) is a vegetable eaten extensively in soups and salads in Greece, Lebanon and other parts of the Mediterranean where the incidence of both heart disease and cancer is low, so it has been suggested that purslane could be cultivated as a source of 18:3 omega-3 from plants rather than seeds from which oils are usually processed.

In summary, doctors are cautious at the present time about any high supplementary consumption of omega-3 fatty acids. There is, at the moment, no good scientific evidence that omega-3s will reverse any *pre-existing* cardiovascular disease, and prolonged consumption of highly unsaturated oils to lower blood lipids may result in a deficiency of vitamin E. Omega-3s increase the risk of gallstone formation and bile-duct disease, and possibly the risk of colon cancer. Women, who already have a lower risk than men for heart disease, but a higher one for bile-duct disease, could find it especially harmful to add omega-3s without reducing overall fat consumption.

And while thinned blood and longer clotting time may benefit the heart and arteries, these conditions can aggravate bleeding due to illnesses such as gastritis, kidney disease and diverticulosis. Anti-clotting properties can also lead to complications such as easy bruising and a profuse longer bleeding time if you have an accident or need an emergency operation.

But not all the evidence is in, and studies in the U.S. have so far been inconclusive. Much more research and investigations need to be done before firm conclusions can be drawn.

WHAT OF THE FUTURE?
Clinical studies are following several avenues of research: Manufacturers of medical imaging systems are exploring the ever-increasing use of computers to develop new machines to give sharper pictures of hearts beating, blood coursing through arteries, and tiny obstructions in veins – magnetic resonance imaging, computed tomography, ultrasound, and positron emission tomography using short-lived radioactive isotopes. Drugs are being constantly reviewed and refined. Cardiologists are using increasingly sophisticated skills to widen heart arteries with tiny balloons (angioplasty) or stainless steel cylinders (stents), or removing plaque from clogged arteries by using minute rotating drills or argon lasers (a procedure called atherectomy); surgeons are performing intricate operations for pacemaker implantation, bypasses and heart transplants. Research programs are gaining a better understanding of the biology of vessel wall injury and the production and removal of lipoproteins.

The next decade will see a massive effort in cholesterol control. Researchers at the Rogosin Institute at New York Hospital, Cornell Medical Center, have been experimenting with a drastic three-hour technique called LDL-pheresis that literally sends your blood out for cleaning, whirls it through a centrifuge and returns it to your body virtually free of fat and cholesterol.

There will be new products in your food supply: scientists at Cornell University working with the University of Wisconsin, Madison, are trying to remove cholesterol from foods such as butter and egg yolks in a technique similar to decaffeinating coffee. And in California, a large egg farm has modified the hens' diet to produce eggs with less cholesterol.

How atherosclerosis develops is still not precisely known, but there is no question that preventing or delaying it is the preferred approach to the control of this disease. Modifying diet to reduce fats and cholesterol will remain the foundation of prevention, and part of post-bypass therapy to minimize further plaque formation.

4

Fats and Cancer

More than 475,000 Americans died of cancer during 1987, with more than 900,000 new cases in that same period. The costs of cancer have been estimated at $72 billion.

Cancer is not just one disease, but a group of more than a hundred different types, all with one common feature of the uncontrolled growth and spread of abnormal cells. Scientists have learned that cancer can develop in the body's cells through a series of separate changes that can take place over a period of years. Many factors can determine if the changes are going to occur. Of prime importance are the genes that you are born with and your family's history of cancer. The day is not far off when you will be able to have a sample of your blood analyzed at a microscopically early stage, long before a tumor is X-ray-visible or before symptoms appear, to check your vulnerability to cancer. The technology is there.

Other factors can be called "environmental," such as whether you smoke, the work you do, the amount of alcohol you drink, and certain types of food you eat. It has been estimated that **35 percent of all human cancers are diet-related**. Cancer-causing agents, *carcinogens*, include certain synthetic and natural chemicals that can be in the air you breathe, in water, diagnostic X-rays, radiation treatment and radioactive isotopes, excessive

78

sunlight and the food you eat. Certain viruses are also suspected of being initiators or promoters of a small number of cancers. The extensive laboratories of the U.S. National Cancer Institute test 50,000 different compounds every year.

Some carcinogens in the environment are difficult to avoid – such as smog, contaminated water and hazardous wastes; but many cancers may be prevented by reducing your exposure to carcinogens just with the personal choices you make. When it comes to cancer, obviously you want to do all you can.

The National Cancer Institute lists some of the things you can do:

- Keep your intake of *all* fats (both saturated and unsaturated) to no more than 30 percent of total calories. Studies suggest that a high intake of dietary fat is a risk factor. Large amounts of PUFAs may promote the growth of tumors.

- Have a variety of food in your daily diet to include generous amounts of fresh whole fruits, vegetables (especially the cruciferous kind), whole grains and wholegrain breads and cereals. Cut back on bacon and charred barbecued meat. Keep calories low enough that you stay trim, since being overweight is another risk factor of certain cancers.

- If you can't do without alcohol, drink only in moderation – no more than one or two drinks a day.

- Don't smoke cigarettes, pipe tobacco or cigars; don't chew tobacco or take snuff.

- Avoid too much sunlight, particularly if you are fair-skinned, by wearing protective clothing and using effective sunscreens. Make sure your eyes are protected during sunning, as prolonged exposure to ultraviolet light over many years can contribute to the premature development of tumors and cataracts.

- Don't ask for an X-ray if your doctor or dentist does not suggest one. If you do need an X-ray, make sure X-ray shields protect other parts of your body. Keep a record of when and where you have X-rays taken.

- If you are prescribed estrogens for menopausal symptoms or birth control, take them only for as long as necessary in the smallest dose.

- Know the health and safety rules at your place of work, and follow them, especially if you think you are close to dangerous chemicals, dusts, fibers and metals such as aniline dyes, arsenic, asbestos, benzene and benzidine, chromium, coke-oven emissions, nickel, radiation and radioactive materials, soots, tars, and polyvinyl chloride. Wear protective clothing and use safety shields when provided.

The National Cancer Institute also warns that if you are exposed to several carcinogens at the same time, the resulting cancer risk may be *multiplied*. For example, if you have a fatty diet and are also a smoker, you have a greater risk than if you merely add the danger from smoking to the hazard of eating a lot of fat.

Dietary items are probably not *direct* carcinogens that initiate abnormal cell growth, but rather the *promoters* of the action of a carcinogen. To quote from *Diet, Nutrition and Cancer* published in 1982 by the U.S. National Research Council: "The weight of evidence suggests that what we eat during our lifetime strongly influences the probability of developing certain cancers . . ." Research still continues on the relationship of cancer with diet; the link is clearly there. The National Cancer Institute endorses the recommendation of the National Academy of Sciences that 30 percent or less of daily calories should come from fat, to reduce the cancer risk, and there should be an increase in fiber-rich foods and foods rich in vitamins A and C, such as dark green and deep yellow vegetables.

Statistical studies, comparing one country with another, report strong consistent links between death rates of breast and colon cancer and a high consumption of total fat and of foods derived from animal sources, especially beef, pork, eggs and milk. Argentinians, for example, who eat more beef than Americans, also exceed Americans in deaths from breast and colon cancer. In Asian countries, on the other hand, where people have a low intake of beef and fatty foods, these forms of cancer are much less frequent. And when Japanese immigrants come to the U.S., where consumption of fat is considerably higher, the pattern of cancer changes, with the immigrants having higher rates of breast, colon and prostate cancer than people of the same age in Japan. Studies of women migrating from Africa and Asia to Israel also show a striking increase in breast cancer, beginning after ten years in that country. Women migrants from Europe or North America to Israel have no comparable change in their already-high breast-cancer death rates, because the Israeli lifestyle is European with little change in food habits. For others, however, the Israeli diet is much higher in fat and represents a significant departure.

One population study reported in 1983 found that people in England and Wales, whose consumption of fat, meat and sugar were sharply reduced during World War II, had a marked reduction of cancer of the breast and colon. After the war, the rates have climbed back to prewar levels.

Similar but less consistent links have been reported with cancers of the prostate, ovary and endometrium (lining of the uterus or womb). By having a lean cuisine, you may reduce your cancer risk; you can also help control your weight, since obesity is another risk factor involving cancers of the breast, uterus, pancreas and gallbladder.

CANCER OF THE BREAST

Breast cancer, like cancers of the uterus and prostate gland, is influenced by the body's hormones. Scientific studies suggest that high levels of dietary fat give rise to elevated blood prolactin concentrations (prolactin is a hormone regulating the production of milk), with a higher prolactin/estrogen ratio that stimulates tumor development in the breasts. Other studies seem to indicate that some substances produced by intestinal bacteria from cholesterol can imitate the action of female hormones, and may promote tumor growth in hormone-sensitive tissues in the breast (and uterus).

Most breast cancers, as well as benign cysts, begin in the lining of the milk ducts or sometimes in the lobules – the clusters of milk-secreting glands. The glandular type produces tiny, hard, pea-like lumps; ductile cancers cannot be detected so easily and have room to expand surreptitiously.

Breast cancer is rare before the age of 30 and becomes more prevalent in later years. Women most likely to have tumors are those with a strong family history of breast cancer. If your mother had it, you have a risk five times higher than normal. The risk of breast cancer rises somewhat if you reached puberty early, or experienced menopause late in life, if you had children late in life, or if you have never had children.

Because breast cancer is associated with a steady diet high in saturated fats, it may be said that all American women are at considerable risk. It is in fact one of the commonest cancers among women, with about *one in ten* developing the disease, most often in their 40s and 50s. The American Cancer Society estimates that 38,000 women in the U.S. died from it in 1985. At the same time, it has been demonstrated that Japanese women, who normally have low-fat foods, have a lower incidence of breast cancer as well as a lower rate of recurrence following cancer operations. Low-fat meals as diet therapy, therefore, may be useful in treatment as well as prevention.

Breast cancer among men accounts for about 1 percent of all cancers among males each year. That so many victims die is attributed to the fact that it is unexpected and usually is not diagnosed until it has progressed too far. According to Canadian researchers, men in families with a high incidence of female breast cancer and other cancers may be at high risk.

Detection and diagnosis
Early detection and treatment is the best approach. Examine your breasts regularly to become familiar with their usual appearance and feel, and how they vary with different stages in your menstrual cycle. After menopause, continue to check your breasts on a regular basis such as the first day of each calendar month. The shape and size of breasts may change throughout

adult life, with nutrition, monthly menstrual cycle, menopause, childbirth, breast-feeding, age, weight change, birth-control pills and other hormone prescriptions. Overall variation in breast size depends on the amount of body fat surrounding and protecting the internal structure. After menopause, breasts usually shed their layer of subcutaneous fat and glandular tissue shrinks.

Bumps, bruises and similar injuries cannot cause cancer. However, treatment for an injury can sometimes lead a doctor to find a cancer that had gone unnoticed.

See your doctor at once if you discover any unusual lump, discharge, dimpling, puckering or crusting around the nipples. Lumpy breasts don't necessarily mean trouble. Eight out of ten breast lumps are not cancerous and may be due to other causes, but only your physician should make the diagnosis. Lumpiness is often the result of the normal ups and downs of female hormones, and after years of repeated hormonal stimulation and subsidence almost all breasts develop some degree of cystic lumpiness. Two recent studies have shown that women with lumpy breasts that are increasingly painful just before menstruation, get considerable relief after changing to a low-fat diet.

Ask your doctor about breast-screening equipment available in your local hospital, medical center or clinic.

Film-screen mammography, X-ray of your breasts, or *xeromammography* which records the X-ray image on special paper, are techniques sufficiently accurate to detect tumors less than 1/4 inch (6mm) diameter when they may be too small to be felt. X-ray machines used for mammography should deliver no more than one rad of radiation per mammogram. Frequent routine mammograms are not recommended for women without symptoms, however, since it is possible that radiation doses over a long period can slightly increase the risk of breast cancer. Mammography is useful if you have cystic fibrous disease or large breasts; neither of these conditions is thought to cause a higher incidence of cancer, but they can make it difficult to spot new lumps. For a biopsy, your doctor may remove a tiny piece of tissue from the breast mass using a hypodermic needle.

Ultrasound is a useful and painless technique as an adjunct to mammography, that projects high-frequency sound waves into the breasts to detect abnormalities.

Thermography, the detection of the heat pattern given off by the skin, is currently under study to determine if it can be used to predict who will get breast cancer.

Trans-illumination or *diaphanography*, using light to illuminate the breasts' interior, may be used experimentally in addition to mammography.

Magnetic resonance imaging, using radio waves to produce three-dimensional body images, is another experimental procedure still being investigated by cancer specialists.

Breast cancer used to mean certain mutilation – and death for most. Now three out of four women with breast cancer can be saved, depending on the stage of the disease; the majority no longer have to lose their breasts. A woman with breast cancer can expect to be treated with surgery, radiation or powerful cancer-killing drugs, alone or in combination, depending on the type of tumor, its location and stage of development. But a diagnosis of cancer does *not* automatically mean a woman must have a radical mastectomy in which the breast, the underlying muscle tissue and lymph nodes and vessels are all removed. A large, well-respected study published in 1985 showed that removing only the cancerous lump and some surrounding tissue (lumpectomy), followed by radiation, worked just as well as a total mastectomy for tumors less than 1 1/2 inch (38mm) in diameter. If breast cancer has not spread to other tissue, the survival rate five years after treatment is close to 100 percent. If the cancer has spread, however, the rate is 60 percent.

CANCER OF THE COLON AND RECTUM
(COLORECTAL CANCER)

Colon cancer is by far the most common type of cancer for which researchers have been able to establish a genetic link. Scientists headed by Dr. Walter F. Bodmer of the Imperial Cancer Research Fund, London, have found that more than 20 percent of colon cancers arise from genetic defects traced to a specific chromosome. This recent discovery may pinpoint the origin of colon cancer in certain cases. Many cancers of the large bowel develop because people have a susceptibility gene and then are exposed to other environmental factors such as high-fat, high-protein, low-fiber foods typical of most urban industrialized countries.

Recent studies have shown the interaction of a fatty diet and the production of bile acids, and also indicate that it is *total* dietary fat, rather than the type of fat, which plays a role in the growth of colon carcinogens. When food is high in fat and cholesterol, bacteria that live in the gastrointestinal tract break down these foodstuffs into substances that can cause cancer. But with a low-fat, high-vegetable diet, the increase in bulk dilutes carcinogens and promoters, and accelerates the movement of undigested food through the colon, so that cancer-causing chemicals have less contact with the bowel lining.

The large bowel, or large intestine, comprising the colon and rectum, is the last portion of your gastrointestinal tract. The colon consists of four sections: the first, called the *ascending* colon, lies on the right side of your abdomen. Making a sharp turn at the liver, the tube becomes the *transverse* colon. A downward turn at the spleen is the beginning of the *descending* colon, which passes into the pelvic area and forms a curving loop called the *sigmoid* colon. At the very end is the *rectum*. Most cancers of the large bowel occur on the left side in the sigmoid section closest to the rectum.

Colorectal cancer occurs more frequently in the United States, Britain, Western Europe, Australia and New Zealand than in Japan, Africa and most of the developing or Third World countries. The American Cancer Society estimated 60,000 deaths in the U.S. in 1987, rates being high in the Northeast and Midwest, and highest in the State of Connecticut. Large-bowel cancer is one of the most common forms of cancer among Americans of both sexes. It is most prevalent in people over 40, with little difference in incidence rates among blacks and whites.

Detection and diagnosis

Symptoms of colorectal cancer are blood in the stool (either bright red or black), changes in bowel habits (such as constipation or diarrhea), abdominal discomfort and pain. Intestinal polyps, or growths in the colon, are believed to be precursors of colorectal cancer, and researchers are trying to develop a blood test that can identify people who have inherited the genetic defect that is responsible for polyposis. The larger the polyp, the more likely it is to be malignant.

Diagnosis by your doctor can involve a number of procedures, including digital examination of your rectum, direct viewing of the rectum and sigmoid section of the colon with instruments called a proctoscope and sigmoidoscope, a barium-enema X-ray examination, and examination of the entire colon with a flexible colonoscope using fiber-optics. A barium-enema X-ray examination will show all significant growths larger than 1/4 inch (6mm). Your doctor will probably make a chemical analysis of a small stool sample for microscopic blood, since most bowel cancers seep a little blood (although the presence of blood in the stool may not necessarily be due to cancer but other conditions such as hemorrhoids). A stool test may also determine whether cells shed from the colon contain defective genetic material as an early warning that a cancer has begun to grow. Chances of survival are higher when the disease is found before it has spread beyond the wall of the colon.

CANCER OF THE PROSTATE

In forty countries, a correlation has been found between prostatic cancer mortality and the per capita consumption of dietary fat.

The prostate gland in the male reproductive system is normally about the size of a walnut, and lies just below the bladder, surrounding part of the canal that empties the bladder. Its function is to produce fluid for semen.

Despite its tiny size and minor duties, the prostate causes distressing symptoms in 75 percent of men over the age of 50. Three basic problems that occur in the prostate are *prostatitis*, an infection of the gland — the most common prostate problem in younger men; *benign prostatic hypertrophy*, an enlargement of the prostate — usually in men over 40; and *prostate cancer.*

Before 1900, prostate cancer was considered a rare disorder. Today it accounts for 18 percent of all male cancer cases. One reason for the increase is that more men are living longer and prostate cancer occurs most frequently in older men, the risk increasing after the age of 50. Rates for black males are greater than those for whites in every age group. The highest death rates are found in the United States, Northern European countries, Australia and New Zealand. The lowest death rates occur in South and Southeast Asian countries.

At a Workshop on Fat and Cancer held at the National Institutes of Health, Bethesda, Maryland, in December 1979, Dr. P. Hill of the American Health Foundation stated "During the last century, dietary patterns have changed in Western society and in Japan, with a marked increase in fat consumption. Concomitantly, the incidence of prostatic cancer (and breast cancer) has increased, with a greater increase in Japanese men and women . . . . In the United States the incidence of prostatic cancer is closely related to the consumption of fat in the form of meat and dairy products." In the United States, an analysis of death rates from 1950 to 1969 showed that prostate cancer occurred in areas where people had high consumption of beef and dairy products. On the other hand, the lower rate of prostate cancer among Seventh-Day Adventists may be related to their lacto-ovo-vegetarian diet, free of meat, poultry and fish, and low in fats.

Detection and diagnosis
While much campaigning has persuaded many women to have regular cervical pap smears and breast exams to detect cancer, there has been no comparable public drive for men over 40 to have yearly rectal exams, even though such examinations are the key to catching prostate cancer in its early, curable stages.

Warning signs include changes in bladder habits, a burning sensation when urinating, or blood in the urine. The majority of men with prostate cancer, however, have no symptoms, so a routine rectal digital examination by a physician is an important annual test after the age of 40. About 50 per cent of prostatic nodules detected by this method are eventually found to be cancerous. A new diagnostic technique which is quick and painless is the use of ultrasound scans to give a visual image of internal organs by reflected sound waves to detect very early prostate cancer.

Dr. Patrick C. Walsh of Johns Hopkins Hospital in Baltimore has devised an operation that removes cancerous prostate glands yet preserves a man's sexual function, retaining potency. Dr. Fernand Labrie of Laval University Medical Center, Quebec, has been successfully treating patients by combining an anti-androgen drug, that cuts off cancer-stimulating secretions from the adrenal gland, with a chemical that blocks hormones secreted by the testicles. This hormone-blocking therapy avoids surgical castration.

CANCER OF THE LIVER

A common problem among alcoholics, the risk of this disease is increased when the liver is constantly overloaded with a buildup of unused fatty acids.

The liver is your body's largest glandular organ. Bile, cholesterol and digestive enzymes are among the vital substances made in the liver in the normal digestive process. Fats increase the production of bile acids, and some bile acids have been observed to act as promoters of tumor growth. The consumption of certain seeds with a high oil content, such as peanuts, is linked to cancers of the liver (also of the stomach and kidney), apparently because of a particular fungus *Aspergillus flavus* which is a parasite of oily seeds. Toxins of this fungus (aflatoxins) have been found to be carcinogenic in laboratory studies of animals.

Secondary liver cancer is a result of the spread of cancer from elsewhere in the body (frequently the breast or colon) not cured by surgery or other treatment.

Detection and diagnosis
Liver cancer produces no obvious symptoms, although in later stages there may be weight loss, loss of appetite, possibly fever and jaundice. For diagnosis, your doctor might call for a liver scan using radioactive substances, or an angiogram using an opaque substance visible on X-rays, or an ultrasound examination. A vaccine that can prevent liver cancer is now available, made with genetically-programmed yeast.

CANCER OF THE PANCREAS
Links between diet and cancer of the pancreas have not yet been extensively explored, but a recent population study conducted in Sweden suggests there may be a connection. Researchers compared intakes of various foods by 99 individuals who had the disease with two sets of control groups. Increased risk was associated with a high frequency of eating grilled and fried meats, fish and other foods, suggesting in this study that the link is not with the food but with the cooking method. Higher risk also corresponded with the consumption of large quantities of margarine, especially among those who admitted using more than a tablespoon on a single slice of bread.

CAN YOU AVERT CANCER WITH FOOD?
So far, no nutritional cancer treatment has been able to halt or reverse cancer, but a good diet may help prevent cancer.

Even though new evidence is still emerging, and many of the studies backed by the National Cancer Institute will not be finished for several years, researchers are already drawing a profile of those individuals who may benefit most from dietary changes. Clinical evidence may show that people already exposed to known or suspected cancer-causing agents or carcinogens can be helped by certain nutrients. Other studies may find that drugs based on these nutrients can slow or block the onset of disease.

The U.S. National Research Council says that the mounting evidence indicating animal fat as a cause for cancer, especially of colon and breast cancer, is so damning that they recommend most people decrease their consumption of fats. Current findings implicate *all* forms of fat; only further research will settle questions about the different types of fat.

But there is no suggestion that fat in food is the *only* dietary factor that may trigger development of certain cancers. The National Cancer Institute is supporting research looking at the combined effects in the diet of many nutrients. For example:

High-fiber diets appear to protect against the effects of eating fat – not the soluble fibers that seem to reduce the risk of heart disease, but the insoluble fibers in fresh whole fruits, vegetables and wholegrain products, such as wholegrain cereals, breads, pasta and brown rice. Scientists are uncertain about how fiber works, but they believe it accelerates the excretion of fat.

A major objective of the National Cancer Institute-backed research is to clarify the benefits of *vitamin A* and *beta-carotene*, a natural substance the body converts into vitamin A. Recent research indicates that vitamin A may help prevent cancer of the colon, stomach, prostate, cervix and breast. Vitamin A and beta-carotene may act to forestall cancer by interfering with the proteins that cancer cells use in reproduction and growth. Other research indicates that beta-carotene that is not converted into vitamin A deactivates oxygen molecules produced by carcinogens and believed to trigger malignant tissue growth. Vitamin A is found in liver, eggs and milk, but the most common source of the vitamin is beta-carotene in leafy green and yellow vegetables, such as carrots, squash, spinach, broccoli and cantaloupe melon. High doses of pure vitamin A can be toxic, however, and eating too many carrots, for instance, can turn your skin yellow. Get what you need from the normal amounts found in food.

Several years ago, scientists discovered that nitrates and nitrites found in processed foods such as bacon and hot dogs, are transformed by the body into nitrosamines, a suspected carcinogen. New research has found that *vitamin C* and *vitamin E* block the formation of nitrosamines. Certain populations whose diets are rich in fruits and vegetables containing these vitamins have a low incidence of cancer of the stomach and digestive tract. So researchers are testing whether food containing vitamin C or E, or vitamin supplement pills, can inhibit the development of colon cancer in patients with a history of developing the type of polyps that are thought to be precursors.

The natural element *selenium* occurs in some foods, such as seafood, meats from certain organs, garlic and grains grown in soils rich in the chemical. Although selenium in high doses can be highly toxic, laboratory studies of cancer cells in test tubes and in animals have shown that certain forms of selenium can block cancer-cell growth. Population studies in the Northeast of the United States suggest that people with low selenium in their diets have higher rates of colon, breast and prostate cancer. Most research at the moment is trying to determine levels at which selenium consumption will not produce toxicity.

5

Fats and Weight Control

Humans are literally fatter than pigs in terms of fat as a percentage of body weight, according to an article in the British journal *Nature*.

Chubby, corpulent, fleshy, obese, plump, portly, pudgy, rotund or stout – there are plenty of ways to describe being too fat. Our present-day society is two-faced: it idolizes the sleek, slender and streamlined, and tends to ridicule or discriminate against stereotypes of fat people. But, paradoxically, society also encourages eating. Even though people have become more health and diet conscious, being overweight has developed into a serious threat to public health. Being too thin is undoubtedly hazardous – national and international food programs have concentrated on undernourished peoples and the problems of malnutrition, but obesity has been the subject of only limited scientific research, and pediatric obesity is a relatively new specialized field in which even less is known.

If you weigh 10 to 19 percent more than your ideal body weight, you are termed "overweight;" at 20 percent or more, you are considered "obese." Approximately 34 million adults – one-quarter of the adult population – are significantly overweight. Obesity in American children under the age of 11 has increased 54 percent in the last 15 years. People are getting more and more fat. Go to any large shopping mall and size up the shoppers. What has contributed to this trend towards obesity?

For eons during which humans were hunter-gatherers, the energy-storage mechanism in the body enabled our ancestors to gorge on a kill and then survive long periods of scarcity between kills, to maintain a physically-demanding lifestyle, and to withstand extreme cold. In gloomy, cold weather, rich fatty foods were not only soothing, but a help in building up a layer of flesh as insulation against winter cold.

Today's conditions in the United States present a different picture, and encourage overeating with –

- An abundance of food, and the ability to afford it. Supermarket shelves are stacked high with rich, fatty machine-made foods and "empty calorie" snacks. Affluence makes it all easily accessible.
- A decrease in physical labor. Mechanization discourages physical activity, with a consequent decrease in hard manual work in industry, on the farm and in the home. A shorter working-day in a five-day work week. Everything is "labor-saving." Labor-saving means bodies need less energy from food. Driving has replaced walking, even for short distances; sports are enjoyed more from the stands than on the playing fields. People are living longer now, with even less activity in later years.
- Effortless heating of homes and work places. Fewer people work outdoors now. Many work in offices and live in heated homes, with little use for the fat calories formerly needed to protect against the outside elements. Heating comes with the flick of a thermostat instead of the swing of an ax.

In the nineteenth century, in times of deprivation, typical diseases were scurvy and rickets; in the twentieth century, in times of affluence, the problem is overeating. Put simply: people are eating too much of the wrong foods while making less and less effort. Today we put more food into our bodies than they need or can use. We are becoming "couch potatoes."

Not everyone feels they want to lose weight: an obese women in authority may think she has an advantage in having an imposing figure; an overweight man, especially if he is short or lacking in confidence, may consider his opinions carry more weight if he has some extra pounds. But there are penalties.

WHAT ARE THE CONSEQUENCES OF BEING TOO FAT?

Obesity is unhealthy, dangerous, and *can* be fatal.

In 400 B.C., Hippocrates wrote that "fat men are more likely to die suddenly than the slender," an observation that is borne out by modern research studies. Obesity is a grave threat to good health, increasing the chances of developing many serious diseases, and robbing people of years of life.

Doctors usually measure obesity as a percentage of weight above the ideal. For example, if you weigh 182 pounds (83kg) but should weigh 165 pounds (75kg), you are 17 pounds (8kg) or 10 percent overweight. Life expectancy for those who are more than 15 percent overweight is reduced in escalating proportion to the degree of obesity. Thus −

Increased Mortality as Related to Obesity

Overweight by:	Increased chance of premature death:
15 to 20 percent	10 percent
25 to 35 percent	30 percent
Over 35 percent	50 percent
100 percent	600 percent

"Morbid obesity" is the medical term to describe people who are either twice their ideal weight or at least 100 pounds (45kg) overweight − a life-threatening condition.

In addition to the general discomfort of carrying extra pounds, and excessive sweating, a number of serious disorders can occur, or be aggravated, because of the underlying problem of being too fat. These include −

Hypertension. About 30 percent of obese people whose body weight is 25 percent above normal high have high blood pressure. The Framingham data indicated a 6mm rise in systolic pressure and a 4mm rise in diastolic pressure for a 10 percent increase in body weight.

Premature heart attack or **stroke** caused by the weight of fat on the chest and an enlargement of the size of the heart or an erratic heartbeat.

High blood cholesterol. This occurs twice as often in the overweight as in the non-overweight, in both adults and children.

Development of cancers of the breast, uterus, endometrium, pancreas and gallbladder in obese women; cancers of the colon, rectum and prostate in obese men. Body fat is thought to be a storehouse for carcinogenic chemicals in men and women.

Diabetes. The risk of diabetes is increased about seven times in the obese. Women with fat deposits on the upper body (neck, shoulders and abdomen) have glucose intolerance more often, higher blood insulin levels and larger fat cells than women with lower-body obesity (at buttocks and thighs). As weight increases, a greater percentage of people become diabetic. Losing weight decreases insulin needs.

Osteoarthritis, from pressure of excess pounds on weight-bearing joints, or arthritic changes that limit movement and exercise necessary for normal bone formation.

Gallstones. The obese have a greater risk – far out of proportion to the non-overweight – of developing gallstones which are generally triggered by a greater production of cholesterol in the liver, resulting in elevated cholesterol levels in the body from a supersaturated bile. Overall, the risk is about twice normal, and particularly prevalent among obese women.

Varicose veins and **blood clots** in the veins of the legs.

Sterility, because of hormone imbalances and menstrual abnormalities; or complications in pregnancy.

Lung problems, with a heavy chest wall restricting breathing and lung volume. If you must undergo anesthesia for surgery, there is an increased likelihood of pneumonia or collapse of the lung. Overweight children seem more prone to chest infections.

Psychological problems as a result of social isolation.

Although not all fat people have these problems, excessive weight can aggravate existing disorders with a depression of immune functions, causing more pronounced symptoms, or their appearance at an earlier age, than in a person of normal weight. Risks linked to excess fat are not just confined to the morbidly obese. Physicians consider that even mild degrees of overweight are hazardous because health problems increase progressively even with small increases above the acceptable weight ranges shown in Table 5, especially for instance in patients already diagnosed as having high blood pressure or diabetes. Conversely, when the overweight reduce to a normal weight range, the benefits of slimming are soon seen in lower blood pressure and blood cholesterol, more normal insulin, and a substantial reduction in the risk of angina and sudden death.

HOW DO YOU BECOME OVERWEIGHT?

Heredity factor. Body types generally fall into three groups: *ectomorphs*, *mesomorphs* and *endomorphs*. Ectomorphs are tall and thin, with narrow bodies and thin arms and legs; they have little fat and are not particularly muscular. Mesomorphs are the strong, muscular types, with little fat on their bodies. Endomorphs are stocky and have round bodies with short necks and limbs; they easily develop fat which is mainly on thighs and upper arms. Of course there are many mixtures of body types, but one of these forms usually predominates.

According to a report in the *New England Journal of Medicine*, a team of Danish and American researchers led by Dr. Albert J. Stunkard, obesity specialist at the University of Pennsylvania School of Medicine, found that children's weights closely paralleled the weights of their parents. In the Danish study, the strongest link was found between mother/daughter; the next strongest was between mother/son. The weights of children also correlated to fathers' weights, but not so strongly.

If one parent is obese, a child stands a 40 percent chance of also being obese; if both parents are obese, a child's risk rises to 80 percent, according to Dr. William Dietz of Tufts University School of Medicine in Boston.

TABLE 5
HOW DO YOU MEASURE UP?
HEIGHT AND OPTIMUM WEIGHT RANGE

Height	Weight Men	Women	Height	Weight Men	Women
ft in	pounds	pounds	meters	kilograms	kilograms
4ft 10in		92 - 121	1.47		41.8 - 55.0
4ft 11in		95 - 124	1.50		43.2 - 56.4
5ft		98 - 127	1.52		44.5 - 57.7
5ft 1in	105 - 134	101 - 130	1.55	47.7 - 60.9	45.9 - 59.1
5ft 2in	108 - 137	104 - 134	1.57	49.1 - 62.3	47.3 - 60.9
5ft 3in	111 - 141	107 - 138	1.60	50.5 - 64.1	48.6 - 62.7
5ft 4in	114 - 145	110 - 142	1.63	51.8 - 65.9	50.0 - 64.5
5ft 5in	117 - 149	114 - 146	1.65	53.2 · 67.7	51.8 - 66.4
5ft 6in	121 - 154	118 - 150	1.68	55.0 - 70.0	53.6 - 68.2
5ft 7in	125 - 159	122 - 154	1.70	56.8 - 72.3	55.5 - 70.0
5ft 8in	129 - 163	126 - 159	1.73	58.6 - 74.1	57.3 - 72.3
5ft 9in	133 - 167	130 - 164	1.75	60.5 - 75.9	59.1 - 74.5
5ft 10in	137 - 172	134 - 169	1.78	62.3 - 78.2	60.9 - 76.8
5ft 11in	141 - 177		1.80	64.1 - 80.5	
6ft	145 - 182		1.83	65.9 - 82.7	
6ft 1in	149 - 187		1.85	67.7 - 85.0	
6ft 2in	153 - 192		1.88	69.5 - 87.3	
6ft 3in	157 - 197		1.91	71.4 - 89.5	

Height without shoes. Weight without clothes.
For women 18 to 25 years, subtract 1 pound for each year under 25.
(Source: *FDA Consumer*, November 1986, adapted from Metropolitan Life
Insurance Company Weight Table)

Previous studies of twins brought up separately suggest that
one-half of fat tissue is probably genetically determined and
one-half due to upbringing. But don't conclude that your weight
problems are "all in the genes" and therefore do nothing. On
the contrary, you need to make extra effort, especially with older
children and teens, to prevent and control obesity. Obesity "in
the family" can often be a matter of "inheriting" unwise eating
and exercise habits. Children usually imitate their overeating
parents, and once this poor eating pattern is established, the
"familial" trend to overweight has unfortunately been passed on

to the next generation. But heredity and sex hormones can determine body frame and where the extra poundage is deposited on your body.

Glandular factors. Fatness is often blamed on "glandular" problems, but overweight caused by disorders of the endocrine glands is exceptionally rare, when, for example, excessive steroid hormones are produced by the adrenal glands. Perhaps only 1 or 2 percent of obese people have a weight problem truly related to metabolism, as in hypothyroidism. (People who must take steroid medication for asthma or allergies often suffer from fluid retention and that in turn causes bloating and unwanted pounds.) If ovaries need to be removed, a woman may tend to gain weight.

Fortunately, obesity caused by hormonal imbalance is relatively easy to treat, and correcting the underlying endocrine disorder usually will resolve the problem, although dieting may be necessary to lose the accumulated fat.

Disability factor. You could have "disability obesity" caused by being bedridden for weeks with an injury, illness or stroke. The inactivity encourages fat to be stored instead of being used, and at the same time you may be using your disability as an excuse for overeating.

Gastronomic factor. You may have "gastronomic obesity" if you love to prepare elaborate meals, indulge in fine wines, and consider yourself a gourmet.

The garbage disposer. You could be a nutritional garbage disposer, nibbling all day long, always cooking, or eating leftover food, making sure "nothing goes to waste." But it goes to your waist!

The basic cause of being overweight is taking in more calories than your body needs. Unneeded calories become large sources of energy stored away as fat in your body. Calories do count! And a key point in weight loss is to change the composition of your food intake by cutting down on dietary fats, which have the highest concentration of calories of anything you eat − or drink.

1 gram of dietary fat gives you about 9 calories. All the usual dietary fats have the same caloric value, which is twice that of proteins or carbohydrates. Why eat large amounts of the very substance — fat — you are trying to lose? Fat in foods has a chemical profile very similar to the fat in your body, so your body absorbs it easily. Eating fat will make you fat.

1 gram of alcohol gives you 7 calories. How many alcoholic drinks do you have each day? They are high in "empty calories" that really add up.

1 gram of protein or carbohydrate gives you 4 calories. How many unnecessary sugary-sweet foods or soft drinks do you have each day? These *simple* carbs are quickly converted to fat deposits. On the other hand the process of turning *complex* carbs such as beans and pastas into body fat is highly complicated; your body must go through many metabolic steps to convert them into fat.

CALORIES AND METABOLISM

Everybody talks about calories — but just what *is* a calorie and what does it do? It's a unit of energy determined by the actual heat produced. Metabolism of food generates energy in the form of heat, and this heat energy is fuel for the body. This is why physical labor makes you hot, and when food metabolism stops after death, the body cools down.

Metabolism is an equation — the sum of all the chemical processes involved in the maintenance of life, especially the growth of new tissue, the repair of tissue, breakdown and elimination of old tissues, and the production of energy. Knowing the calorie content of food is useful in balancing energy intake and outgo.

Your *Basal Metabolic Rate (BMR)* is the rate at which you use energy to maintain body temperature, heartbeat, breathing and muscle tension, when you are sleeping or in a resting state. It is slightly higher in men than in women; it is higher in childhood, with increases during growth spurts such as puberty, during pregnancy and lactation. It varies with the amount of caffeine you have and if you are a smoker. Generally, the BMR for an average healthy man is between 1600 and 1800 calories per day, and for an average woman, between 1200 and 1400. A normal decline in your metabolic rate, of about 15 percent, occurs between the ages of thirty and eighty. It is still uncertain whether obese people have a lower-set BMR that might explain their condition.

You can easily calculate your own individual caloric needs: first, divide your weight in pounds by 2.2 to convert it to kilograms. Average BMR is 1 calorie per kilogram of body weight per hour; so your daily BMR is 1 calorie x weight x 24 hours. Then calories needed for physical activity must be added to this figure. As a rough guide to the calories you need for activity, add –

20 percent if you are very sedentary.
30 percent for sedentary people (secretaries, drivers, professionals).
40 percent if you are moderately active (most industrial workers, mailpersons, waiters/waitresses).
50 percent for the very active (construction laborers, farm workers, dockers).

For example:
A man weighing 154lb (70kg); 70 x 24   = 1680 calories (BMR)
Moderately active: 1680 x 40%   =   672 calories
Daily total should be: 1680 + 672   = 2352 calories

A woman weighing 132lb (60kg); 60 x 24 = 1440 calories (BMR)
Sedentary occupation: 1440 x 30%   =   432 calories
Daily total should be: 1440 + 432   = 1872 calories

As a general rule, in order to get sufficient essential nutrients, an adult man should not have less than 1600 calories, a teenage boy should not dip below 1800 or 2000, an adult woman (neither pregnant nor nursing) not less than 1200, and a teenage girl not less than 1400 to 1600 calories.

Out of your total daily calorie needs, you will want to allocate only a limited proportion of fat calories, as shown in Table 6.

TABLE 6
CALORIES AND FAT PERCENTAGES

Total daily calories	Recommended for:		Percentage of fat					
			10%	20%	25%	30%*	35%	40%
1400	Women 45+	Calories	140	280	350	**420**	490	560
		Grams of fat	16	31	39	**47**	54	62
1600	Women 18-44	Calories	160	320	400	**480**	560	640
		Grams of fat	18	36	44	**53**	62	71
1800	Girls 12-17	Calories	180	360	450	**540**	630	720
		Grams of fat	20	40	50	**60**	70	80
2000	Children 6-11 and men 55+	Calories	200	400	500	**600**	700	800
		Grams of fat	22	44	56	**67**	78	89
2400	Men 18-54	Calories	240	480	600	**720**	840	960
		Grams of fat	27	53	67	**80**	93	107
2600	Boys 12-17	Calories	260	520	650	**780**	910	1040
		Grams of fat	29	58	72	**87**	101	116

* Recommended maximum.
Note: 28 grams of fat = approximately 1 ounce or 2 tablespoons.

The single most important non-genetic factor that determines whether or not you have a sluggish metabolism is the size of your muscles. The more muscle tissue you have, the more calories you burn. Dietitians estimate an average Olympic athlete needs 6000 calories per day. When food is not fully metabolized into its end products of carbon dioxide and water, it is stored as fat, which represents a stored fuel that can be used for energy if and when needed, much like gasoline in the tank of a car. An active large-boned person, living in a severely cold climate, needs more energy derived from food than a less active small-framed person living in a warm environment. Polar explorers and native people in Arctic regions pulling sleds may need 5000 calories a day — even up to 8000 calories — with high-fat foods such as pemmican (dried meat mixed with lard).

If you are making deposits of fat, you are storing too many calories for your level of activity. This does not necessarily mean you are eating too much food – but the wrong *type* of food such as fat that concentrates calories in a small portion. Or it may be that you are getting too little exercise if you are desk-bound, tied to a computer, glued to your kitchen chair, or watching television and video for hours (the couch potato). The consequences can be measured in belt notches. Although housework and looking after young children can be tiring, don't assume they provide all the activity you need. Housework is real work but not a calorie-burner, because most chores are fairly brief and soon interrupted. To burn a sizable number of calories, you need to keep muscles at work continuously for at least half an hour – a brisk walk, a bicycle ride or a swim.

While some people are fat because they overeat or under-exercise, or both, studies show that many overweight people do not eat more than normal-weight people do, and some eat less. The difference lies in your body's ability to burn up the calories you consume instead of putting a high proportion into storage as body fat. One theory of weight control suggests you may be an "underburner" – someone whose body tends to store food as fat instead of converting it to heat and burning it off. Underburners are more, not less, energy-efficient than their thin counterparts, with their bodies running so well that they get incredible mileage out of the smallest number of calories; they conserve energy. If you are one of these underburners, you may have to try harder to keep within your weight range. Cutting fat calories and exercising more will make it easier. But with the cells of your body slowing down as you age, if you eat like you always have done – by the time you reach 50 you will probably weigh far more than you should.

HOW FAT IS TOO FAT?

As most studies are based on body weight, Table 5 shows the U.S. Metropolitan Life Insurance Co. height/weight tables for young adults. No adjustments were made for teens or the increasing number of people over 60, so the implication is that you should stay within your weight range all through your adult life. You need to set yourself a practical goal by deciding what weight range would be healthy for you – one that you can realistically reach and maintain. (Remember that being ultra-thin also has its hazards.) Since most people tend to gain weight in their thirties, forties and fifties, the ideal is to hold the line against a spreading midsection or try to maintain the weight you were at about the age of 25. Some women may lose height in later years if vertebrae fracture with osteoporosis.

To find out if you need to lose weight, stand in front of a mirror and jog in place; does anything shake that shouldn't? Weight doesn't always reflect obesity; what counts is not always what the bathroom scales read or even what the mirror reflects. Two men of the same age and same weight can have different proportions of obesity if, for instance, one is an office worker and another is a lumberjack. Thin people don't always have a low percentage of body fat, nor do large persons always have a high proportion. And as you age, maintaining the same weight does not mean necessarily that you have maintained the best ratio of fat tissue to lean tissue.

In clinical research, the *Quetelet* or *Body Mass Index* (*BMI*) is often used as an approximate measure of adult body fatness. It is a single number describing the relationship between height and weight. The calculation is simple: weight in kilograms divided by the square of height in meters (Wt.kg/Ht.m^2). A BMI of 22.5 or slightly less is considered normal for a man corresponding to the midpoint of weight for a person of medium frame on the Metropolitan height/weight tables. A BMI of 24.8 is 10 percent above desirable weight, indicating overweight; and a figure of 27.2 is 20 percent over, and considered obese. However, extremely well-exercised athletes may have an excess weight in relation to height, and therefore a BMI that indicates they are overweight – but that weight is related to muscle, and they would not be overfat.

There are several methods of making an evaluation of body composition. One method is *hydrostatic weighing* while being immersed in water, often used in training gyms and weight-loss clinics by athletes and others interested in finding out their fat-lean ratio. This procedure does not actually measure body fat but body density, and this density figure is then translated into percentage fat. Some health clubs may use *sound waves* to pick up density differences between muscle and fat; or *electrical impedance units* that work on measurement of electrical resistance (current passes slower through fat than it does through lean tissue). Electrodes are attached to hand and foot, a mild current is passed through the body, from which a percentage of body fat can be calculated. Other methods include *neutron activation* (measuring carbon in the body, as an indicator of fat), and *light interaction* (using near-infrared light in a wand pressed to the middle of the biceps).

Measurement of the width of the fat layer directly beneath the skin is another method which takes into account the fact that subcutaneous tissue is a repository of fat. Physicians concerned with weight reduction and physical conditioning use pincer-like devices called *calipers* to measure the thickness of skinfolds at shoulder blade, front of thigh and triceps muscle. Skinfold thickness can then be translated accurately into terms of percentage of body fat.

But you can give yourself the "pinch test," by tensing your left arm and pinching skin at the back of your arm between thumb and forefinger; if you can pinch more than an inch, you are probably carrying more weight than you should be. Feel for the accumulation of fat stores at waist and hips.

Hormonal differences between the sexes affect body composition, with men generally having more muscle and less fat than women. This in turn influences the rate at which calories are burned. Muscle tissue is more active metabolically and burns calories at a faster rate than fat tissue does.

Exactly how much body fat is ideal is a matter of slight dispute among exercise physiologists and other experts. The following body-fat standards for athletes were set up by the National Athletic Health Institute in Inglewood, California:

Ideal Percentage of Body Fat

Age	Men	Women	Age	Men	Women
16	12%	18%	37-39	19%	25%
17-19	13%	19%	40-43	20%	26%
20-23	14%	20%	44-46	21%	27%
24-26	15%	21%	47-49	22%	28%
27-29	16%	22%	50-53	23%	29%
30-33	17%	23%	54+	24%	30%
34-36	18%	24%			

But for non-athletes, according to Fit or Fat Systems in Portland, Oregon, a healthy average maximum of body fat for men of all ages would be 15 percent, and a healthy maximum for women of all ages 22 percent. Due to bone-density differences, black men should strive for body fat of 12 percent, black women 19 percent, Asian men 18 percent and Asian women 25 percent. However, if you have a history of being overweight or a genetic predisposition to hold on to fat, it may be difficult if not impossible to achieve these ideals.

WHERE DO YOU STORE FAT?

Recent evidence from several countries suggests that *where* you store fat may be more important than how fat you are. So-called "male type" obesity – the bulging abdomen sometimes known as "beer belly" or "executive spread" – seems to present more of a threat than fat lower down around the hips and buttocks ("female type" obesity). Bulging bellies appear to increase the risk of developing cardiovascular disease and diabetes. Ideally a man's waist should measure at least six inches less than his chest. Bring out your tape measure! For every inch your waistline exceeds the size of your chest, you can deduct two years from your life expectancy. Or give yourself the ruler test: lie on your back and balance a ruler lengthwise along the middle of your body. Between your rib cage and the top of your pelvis your abdomen should be flat. If the ruler slants upward, it's an indicator of excess fat. Why is abdominal fat worse? Researchers speculate that fat cells there may be more metabolically active, perhaps pumping more fat into the bloodstream.

Incidentally, there is no such thing as "cellulite," a term coined in European salons and spas, and used by many people when referring to the dimpled fat deposited under the skin on a woman's hips and thighs that seems to stubbornly resist diet and exercise. Although the American Medical Association has taken no official position on this subject, the *Journal of the American Medical Association*, June 21, 1976, stated "There is no medical condition known or described as cellulite in this country." Then what is it?

Women are biologically programmed to have fat reserves at thighs, buttocks and hips for childbearing, nursing and, after menopause, the storage of the hormone estrogen. Female estrogen influences this fat deposition, but the fat in these places is no different from the fat anywhere else in the body. Bands of ligaments or fibrous tissue run from the skin through the fat, attach to the underlying muscles and deeper tissue layers, and separate the fat cell compartments. When you have a lot of body fat, the fat cells increase in size, apparently causing the compartments of fat to bulge and push up against the skin, while the ligaments pull down the skin – hence the skin looks waffled or dimpled.

If cellulite were really different from other fat, some chemical or structural variation should be evident, but this is not the case. Dr. Neil Solomon, former Secretary of Maryland's Department of Health and Mental Hygiene, conducted a double-blind study with 100 people at Johns Hopkins University and City Hospital in Baltimore, in an attempt to differentiate cellulite from common fat. Needle biopsies were taken from people with dimpled, lumpy, fatty tissue resembling what pill promoters call cellulite, as well as from people without cellulite. When pathologists were asked to compare the samples, there were no differences under the microscope – they all looked like ordinary fat cells.

Two German physicians writing in the *Journal of Dermatologic Surgery and Oncology* (March 1978) about their study of so-called cellulite, found certain characteristics in women's skin and underlying tissue that probably explain why women exhibit the phenomenon and men generally don't: the connective tissue beneath women's skin creates fat-cell chambers that are large and round, while in men the chambers are divided into small, polygonal units that don't readily bulge when filled. In addition, certain outer layers of skin in women are thinner than in men, and more likely to reveal any bulging of fat cells underneath.

Many women are simply not biologically designed for the modern, lean body-line. Not everyone can look like Brooke Shields, and some shouldn't try. Bodies designed by genes don't always fit designer jeans.

Unfortunately many people are lured by advertisements promoting heating pads, reducing belts, creams, pills or sponges that "work like magic" to "take away the cellulite;" tablets are offered that consist of vitamins, minerals and herbs possibly with diuretic properties causing a temporary loss of water to make the body appear slimmer. Enzyme injections in beauty salons have been shown, in scientific studies, to be no more effective than a placebo. The only area where you will be sure to lose weight is in your wallet!

Obesity experts agree that no equipment, exercise or treatment is capable of spot-reducing — removing fat exclusively from a single area of your body. The only way to have thinner thighs is to reduce fat from all over your body and to reduce the amount of fat in your food. Fatty foods go straight to fat cells.

THE "ORGAN" OF OBESITY
In recent years, scientists have learned much about the "organ" of obesity — adipose tissue.

In research at Harvard University and other centers, neurophysiologists have shown that appetite is regulated by a delicate mechanism in the *hypothalamus*, a small cluster of specialized cells at the base of the brain. When you sniff aromas through your nostrils, or receive them between nasal passages and mouth when eating or drinking, olfactory receptors convey messages to the *limbic* region of the brain. The limbic system activates the hypothalamus (the master switchboard for the pituitary gland) to stimulate the production of hormones controlling appetite, body temperature, metabolism, caloric levels, and much more. The *appestat*, or appetite regulator, monitors levels of fat, protein, sugar and oxygen in the blood, and reacts to chemical signals from the digestive system. With sufficient exercise, the appestat balances caloric intake and outgo so precisely for many people that their weight hardly varies by more than a pound within a year. But if you have a sedentary lifestyle, your appestat works less effectively and then you may be eating more than you should. According to nutritionist Dr. Jean Mayer, exercise that strengthens the heart muscle will not only burn off excess fat but will also reset the appestat to function better, helped by adjustments in the type and amount of food that you eat.

A fat, or adipose cell (*adipocyte*), is made up of adipose tissue and water, in different proportions, with these proportions changing throughout life. Adipose cells are not as sluggish as you may think, but capable of a high rate of metabolism. Like tiny balloons which can be inflated and deflated according to need, the proportion of fat to water in cells increases as they store excess fat and decreases as fats are used up. Studies indicate that babies in the first few months of life can have substantial increases in fat cell size.

The total number of fat cells in your body is fixed by the time you are in your late teens, with the actual number varying with the individual. If an infant is overfed, the *number* of fat cells can increase substantially (two to five times normal) in the still-developing adipose tissues, and once these cells become established, the number will not decrease in later life, despite weight reduction efforts. Although not absolutely inevitable, the puppy fat of youth can lead to overweight in the teenage years, and an increased risk of having a lifetime of obesity. But if weight gain occurs when you are an adult, it is due to an increase in the *size* rather than the number of fat cells. The proportion of fat to water inside the fat cell changes, and the fat cell will consist mainly of fat. If you try to lose weight as an adult, the fat cells decrease in size but the number of fat cells will always be constant. Researchers have been investigating the mechanisms which determine the composition of adipose cells, particularly the cellular "sodium pump" system regulating the amounts of sodium and potassium governing the retention of water. Scientists are now confirming the presence of a calorie-burning mechanism which is in charge of burning up extra calories: a certain kind of fat called "brown adipose tissue" (BAT) or "brown fat," lying around the back of the neck and along the backbone. This tissue, which is activated by the hypothalamus, is apparently more abundant in adults who are exposed to the cold. When this mechanism is working incorrectly, extra calories are turned into fat, and apparently BAT activity tends to be very low in overweight people.

FADS AND FALLACIES

Probably no other aspect of health is surrounded by such a mixture of facts, fads and fallacies as obesity, weight reduction and the fight against flab. The weight-loss industry bristles with ingenious inventions: the fork that lights up when it is overloaded with too much food; a $25 headband that you plug in before meals to promote negative thoughts about food; an $80 suit that you wear filled with crushed ice and water to increase metabolism. Body wraps, sauna belts, machines that provide electrical jolts to muscle, and even ear acupuncture — all have been promoted as ways to fight flabbiness. Steam baths and saunas promise to "melt pounds away;" vibrator belts invite you to shake off unwanted fat. Quick-weight-loss books are often on the best-seller lists even though they offer conflicting advice on how to lose lard. In the long run, no fad diet really works.

The Water, Grapefruit, and Low-Carbohydrate Diets claim to make you pounds thinner overnight. The Atkins and Scarsdale Diets are overloaded with fats and cholesterol, and many others are downright dangerous with their nutrition imbalance which can start you on the road to eating disorders. One-food diets can never supply enough nutrients to keep you healthy, even with vitamin supplements. Some desperate dieters have risked and sometimes lost their lives through drastic slimming formulas, pills, potions and weight-loss procedures such as bulimic purging.

Many people practice "morning anorexia" − no breakfast, a light lunch, then a heavy meal at night, overloading on fat and calories when they least need them.

Slimming diets used for only short periods of time are often futile. In many cases, after losing 5 or 10 pounds, dieters go back to old patterns of eating, and any temporary loss is soon regained. Two-thirds of all slimmers go off diets in about 60 days. The all-too-common "yo-yo" cycle of weight loss followed by gain may leave you worse off than before you started: when an obese person starts scaling down, repeated weight losses and gains can trigger the development of gallstones, with a chemical derangement in the liver producing a high concentration of cholesterol in the bile.

Starvation diets, stopping all nutrition except juices and water, can be dangerous, unless closely medically supervised, particularly if you have heart disease, liver disease or gout. Fasting does not "remove toxins," purify or "rest" your metabolic system. Instead, it puts unnecessary stress on your body to operate without enough fuel, and can result in the loss of important body protein, potassium and calcium. If your doctor does decide on this method for you to lose weight, it should be carried out in hospital, to monitor carefully any problems with your heart, blood pressure or acute gout.

Very-low-calorie diets refer to slimming on less than 800 calories daily. Designed for use in certain cases of extreme obesity, they require strict supervision of doctor and dietitian and are not do-it-yourself diets. They can be especially dangerous if you are pregnant, a teenager, a child, or a diabetic. They may be deficient in essential nutrients and can be associated with dizziness, nausea, fatigue, dehydration, electrolyte imbalance, increased uric-acid levels and acidosis. Complications can result in damage to your liver, kidneys and heart, and can trigger arthritis.

Protein-sparing modified fasts provide 200 to 400 calories from protein daily in order to prevent the body from breaking down its own muscle tissue to meet its protein needs. Despite this claim, muscle mass is not preserved. The original liquid protein diets which use a poor quality, hydrolyzed protein can pose special dangers including sudden death, heart irregularities and metabolic imbalances during the period of semi-starvation.

Low-carbohydrate high-protein diets claim to cause the body to burn fat for energy and produce "ketone bodies" (a state of *ketosis*) which must be excreted in the urine. The excretion of ketone bodies does not "wash away" significant amounts of calories. If you lose weight on a ketonic diet, it is primarily because your body loses water and not fat tissue, and this diet ignores the need to reduce dietary fats. Low-carbohydrate diets limit fruit, vegetables and grains, and can lead to vitamin and mineral deficiencies. A high proportion of protein in the diet puts a strain on kidneys to get rid of excess end-products of protein metabolism.

Diuretics and laxatives trigger loss of water weight, not body fat. They can cause dehydration and electrolyte imbalances. Excessive use of laxatives can impair bowel function and interfere with vitamin and mineral absorption, and thus hormone production and bone metabolism.

Diet pills, appetite suppressants, amphetamines and related drugs may be effective for only three to six weeks. These drugs can raised blood pressure, cause insomnia, and in large doses, severe mental disturbances. You can become psychologically addicted to amphetamines, and they should only be used when prescribed and closely supervised by your doctor, especially if you have hypertension, heart disease or are nervous. Your physician may prescribe mazindol, diethylpropion, fenfluramine or phentermine, which can be helpful in the short term but they can create troublesome side effects such as nausea, mouth dryness, diarrhea and sometimes depression. Emphasis on drugs, rather than on correcting eating habits, does more harm than good. Many nonprescription slimming tablets are accompanied by dietary guidelines, however, and it is this redirection of eating patterns rather than the pills or drugs themselves that can make the greatest contribution to lasting weight loss.

When body weight is at least 100 pounds (45kg) above normal, or in cases of morbid obesity, drastic approaches are sometimes necessary. If such extreme overweight does not respond to conventional methods and is not due to a treatable endocrine abnormality, doctors may consider jaw-wiring, stomach-stapling, or intestinal-bypass surgery. Initially, jaw-wiring seems to produce considerable weight loss initially with few side effects, but when wiring is removed, weight is often regained rapidly. In the long run, it doesn't seem to be effective, considering the discomfort of the procedure. Stomach-stapling reduces stomach capacity, and an intestinal-bypass operation creates malabsorption because foods bypass most of the small intestine where calories would be absorbed by the body in the ordinary way. Such complex surgical procedures may have undesirable side effects such as severe diarrhea, vomiting, vitamin and calcium deficiencies, kidney stones, gallstones and accumulation of fat in the liver. Sometimes complications can be so serious that the stomach or intestine must be reconnected and brought back to its normal function – with probably a subsequent return to weight gain.

Increasing numbers of men as well as women are undergoing expensive suction-assisted *lipectomy*, usually performed by plastic surgeons for cosmetic reasons. The procedure involves using a curette with a vacuum pump to suck excess fat from thighs, buttocks, abdomen and face to reshape contours. But liposuction is not for the obese, because most doctors put a limit of 4 to 5 pounds (2kg) total that can safely be removed per procedure. When a doctor suctions out fat, he is also removing blood and body fluids; extracting too much without replacing blood supply can result in death. There can be problems of bruising and soreness, excessive bleeding, blood clots, infections and the risks attached to anesthesia. Liposuction is no substitute for proper diet and exercise, and does nothing to correct the underlying habits of overeating which created the extra stores of fat in the first place. Eat like a horse after you have undergone a liposuction operation, and your body will find a place elsewhere to store fat.

A SENSIBLE LIFETIME PLAN

How do you get out of the failed-diet trap? Unfortunately there is no simple, quick and safe solution to weight reduction. You didn't gain extra fat stores overnight, so you can't expect to lose them overnight. It is a long-term project that may take months, and no one method will work satisfactorily for everyone. In any case, if you are more than 30 pounds (13.6kg) overweight and find it impossible to stop gorging, you need the help of a professional. Don't attempt any drastic substantial weight-loss regimen unless you are under the direction of your doctor or dietitian.

Remember that weight loss and fat loss are not identical. Body cells contain water and other nutrients as well as fat, and in the first days of any reducing diet, the dropping numbers on the bathroom scale represent loss of water, not fat. Water loss will depend in part on the proportion of fat, protein and carbohydrate in the diet, and partly on salt intake and other factors that affect body fluids.

A well-planned slimming program, with a gradual change in your lifetime habits of eating, can do much to reduce health risks and increase your likelihood of a longer, more comfortable life. The more successful slimming diets are based on –

1. Keeping an eating diary to get a clear picture of what, when and how much you are eating, snacking and drinking.
2. Adding up the total calories from food, and the calories from fat, keeping the fat ratio to less than 30 percent. There is no easier way to reduce calories in your diet than to eat less fat.
3. Cut out alcohol to cut calories fast.
4. Increasing the fiber content of meals, with healthy fresh unpeeled fruits to satisfy appetite and give a feeling of fullness without fat. Many fibrous foods take longer to chew, forcing you to eat more slowly, and give time for the brain to register satisfaction before you over-consume calories.

5. Cooking (or ordering in a restaurant) no more food than you can eat.

6. Sitting at a table, even if you are only having a small snack, to raise your awareness of putting food into your mouth. Eat slowly to savor each bite, with moderate portions and no seconds! Use small plates and don't serve buffet style.

7. Having a good breakfast, not going to work feeling hungry, and not eating after 8 p.m. (or at least three hours before bedtime).

8. Having several small meals a day — even as many as six mini-meals — if you prefer to eat that way. Numerous studies of weight loss have shown that this can be far better for body and mind than stuffing down one or two big ones.

9. Exercising regularly to consume calories, speed metabolism and firm tissues. Fill your weekend with activities that are action-oriented and not centered around food.

10. Weighing yourself once a week — not daily.

First, you need to have a turn around from calorie excess to calorie deficiency, forcing your body to burn up some of its own materials to provide the energy for its vital activities. Eventually, this calorie deficit is made up by energy obtained mostly from the break down of fat deposits. Fatty tissue gradually shrinks, and body weight continues to decrease as long as you maintain a calorie deficit.

For permanent results, you need a permanent change in food habits — not an unfamiliar daily menu that you find difficult or boring to follow for more than a couple of weeks, but a sensible modification of your own food preferences, with a significant reduction in calories from fats.

Remember, a pound of body fat represents about 3500 calories, so if your daily calorie intake has 500 fewer than usual, you should normally lose about a pound each week (since 500 x 7 = 3500).

Ideally, you should lose weight at a slow but steady rate of no more than two pounds (1kg) each week until you achieve a reasonable goal considering your height and age. For safe, effective and lasting weight loss, the American Dietetic

Association now says that a person should not go below 10 calories per pound of body weight. For example, if you weigh 150 pounds (68kg), you should eat no fewer than 1500 calories per day. This way you are more likely to keep weight off for good. However, this rule doesn't necessarily apply to the morbidly obese who weigh twice the ideal.

Remember the equation: eat less + exercise more = weight loss. Half the battle of the bulge is won by exercise.

As a general rule, when you lose weight, 70 percent is assumed to be fat, and 30 percent is assumed to be muscle, mineral or anything other than fat. When you increase exercise while on a slimming diet, the weight you lose is mostly fat. If you take a brisk walk for 30 minutes every day, you will use more calories, speed up weight loss, improve your cardiovascular fitness, and start to feel *good*! For big men and women, embarrassed about their size, an increasing number of exercise classes cater exclusively to their special needs. See Appendix II for ways to burn up calories.

Incidentally, don't be tempted to start smoking in order to lose weight. Although smokers generally weigh less than nonsmokers, they have a greater health risk. Many smokers, after giving up the habit, tend to have a weight gain of about 20 percent because of increased appetite, improved senses of taste and smell, change in metabolism, and possibly in eating habits. This weight increase is often used by other smokers trying to justify their refusal to quit. But the hazards from smoking outweigh the problems of being heavy or even marginally obese. If you are overweight and a smoker, lose the smoking habit first, then lose weight. However, weight gain doesn't have to be inevitable if you resolve to exercise more − to treat your bloodstream to lungs full of good fresh air − and cut out greasy foods and snacks.

Enlist the support of your family, spouse, roommate or partner. A slimmers' group such as Weight Watchers may help to get you going in the right direction; your local Recreation Department or Y.M.C.A. may offer weight-loss classes. Choose a diet plan that has flexibility in meal planning, with adequate servings from a variety of foods, but which limits fats, sweets and alcohol. Ask yourself: "Is this a sensible eating plan I can follow for the rest of my life?"

PREVENTION – THE EIGHT STAGES IN LIFE

1. **Babies.** The best start to life is breast milk, which on average contains 40 to 50 percent of the calories as fat. Eating habits are formed in infants as soon as they begin taking solid foods. After weaning, at about four months until the age of two, pediatricians believe the total percentage of fat in the diet should still approximate that found in human milk. In the first two years while growth rate is maximum, you want to make sure your baby has a normal growth rate, without producing obesity or malnutrition. Babies need the calories in fat for growth, activity and development of their nervous systems. But after the second year, the American Academy of Pediatrics recommends that fat calories should be between 30 and 40 percent. Between the ages of two and five years children do not grow nearly as rapidly as before, and may need less food for energy. Watch for early obesity. It is important that children should not become overweight; their condition is best determined by the pediatrician, family doctor, or health professional at the local clinic – not just by parents. Too many jars of baby food or bottles of milk will result in a chubby baby and perhaps an obese child as well. Many mothers mistakenly think that large, plump children are always stronger and healthier; or perhaps encourage children to overeat because they themselves have known hunger in the past, but by doing so, parents may be laying the groundwork for an unhealthy life in the future. At the same time, a very low-calorie diet for infants can stunt growth, decrease muscle mass and, in a very young child, adversely affect the brain.

The older an obese child is, the more likely obesity will persist. The goal should be to allow children to grow into a more normal weight, gradually thinning as they become taller – but not all children grow out of their puppy fat. Prevention of obesity in the first place is much more desirable and effective than treating the condition once it is established and poor food habits are deeply ingrained. Don't push food. When children begin to serve themselves they may take more than they need or can reasonably finish; part of their learning experience should be to stop eating when they are satisfied. It can sometimes be a mistake to urge them to eat food items in any particular order or to "clean up their plates." In that way, children learn that eating more food than they really need is a way to please you, and that habit can start a pattern of overeating. Don't use food as a bribe or reward for good behavior or withhold it as a penalty. Carefully monitor the fat and sugar content of meals and snacks.

Experts insist that parents should never tell children they are fat. If one child gets chubby, the whole family can have carefully portioned low-fat meals rather than single out the individual child who may feel a diet is a punishment.

Studies have observed that obese children are generally inactive, so make sure your youngsters walk to school if possible, or ride bicycles, take part in school sports, and have plenty of active games in their spare time, to promote healthy activity. Check that schools have good athletic programs. Ration TV time. The whole family can go for walks together, play tag, kick around a football, play tennis or swim – anything but sitting in the car or watching TV.

2. **Adolescents**. A fat teenager has far less chance of outgrowing obesity than a fat four-year-old. If you have teens at home (or if you yourself are a teenager), you know it is a time of dynamic change. Adolescents achieve 50 percent of their adult body weight and 15 to 20 percent of their adult height during these years. Consequently, teens need additional nutrients to grow and develop to their maximum potential and to feel and look their best. Growth and activity vary so much between individual teenagers that there can be wide differences in caloric and nutrient needs, and erratic eating. Parents may need the help of the family doctor to assess adolescent weight gain. Heavier girls reach puberty at maybe ten or eleven, and as breasts and hips become fuller, many girls tend to see these changes in terms of "getting fat." The sex hormone estrogen encourages fat storage,

and for some teens, signs of their emerging sexuality can make them panic. Food binges can be a way of hiding, or some young people *think* they are too fat when in fact they are extremely thin with problems of anorexia. But by the time they reach twenty, *half* of adolescents in America tend to be too heavy. Active sports and exercise can control weight of girls and develop muscle mass in boys: swimming, skating, tap dancing – whatever they enjoy.

For adolescents to have the necessary vitamins, minerals and other nutrients, they need moderate portions from a variety of foods from the major food groups, but a limit on fat. Make a family rule of "no seconds" on meat servings (if you eat meat) or high-fat food items, but no limit on extra portions of vegetables. Insist that food be eaten in only one or two places in the house (the kitchen and dining room, for instance) and don't allow eating in bedrooms, while watching television or doing homework. Many teens nibble snacks between meals, so keep fresh fruits and raw vegetable sticks ready for munching; with plenty of healthy snacks on hand, your teens won't feel deprived. Show your disapproval of chips and greasy commercial "fast foods."

Suggest to school-meal organizers that menus should offer low-fat choices and home economics courses should include low-fat food preparation. With a new set of low-fat rules incorporated into everyday eating, you can teach your youngsters new options and attitudes about food to last them a lifetime.

3. **Young adults**. Working men and women often need to have meals away from home. Talk with the manager of the company cafeteria or staff restaurant about providing more low-fat dishes on the menus. Try to avoid fast-food chains. If your work is not manual, you don't need those high-fat highly caloric meals. Better still, bring your own healthy low-fat lunch and snacks from home: plenty of fresh fruit, wholegrain breads, crisp raw vegetables and nonfat yogurt. If you're at home with the children, don't snack whenever the youngsters do, as their needs are different from your own. Don't eat dinner twice – once with the children and later with your spouse.

Many women during their menstrual cycles experience weight gain and water retention, fluctuating with the different levels of their female hormones. It is common to have changes of appetite and increased hunger after ovulation and before menstruation when estrogen levels are high. Tune into your body's variations, and try to limit intake of fats, table salt, sweets and alcohol during premenstrual days. If you are prescribed birth-control pills, or the new vaginal rings that release hormones, you may have weight gain depending upon the estrogen strength of the prescription, so diet has to be carefully watched.

4. **Athletes**. Many athletes believe that a thick steak is a good pregame meal because meat makes muscle. Sports physicians disagree. Meat is a poor source of quick energy because it is too high in fat to give you peak performances. Digesting fat is actually an energy drain, so red-meat protein is the least efficient energy source. Fats and oils can cause a lowering of the bloodstream's oxygen-carrying capacity and reduce your sports abilities. Glycogen stores, which provide fuel for the muscles to work, are better supplied by complex carbohydrates such as fruits, vegetables, whole grains and dried beans, peas, etc. − not by fat or protein.

5. **Pregnant mothers**. What you eat before you become pregnant is important, and you may need to plan ahead to achieve a healthy body weight.

If you are underweight, with inadequate body fat, you may have to gain weight before ovulation can take place, since body fat plays a vital role in the production and storage of estrogen, the hormone crucial for ovulation.

If you are overweight, conception may be difficult, and obesity can cause many complications making a normal delivery difficult. One in five American women gains too much weight during pregnancy and then has trouble taking it off. Don't attempt to slim during pregnancy unless you are under the close guidance of your doctor or health adviser at the prenatal clinic. If you have a substandard weight gain while expecting, you are more likely to have a smaller baby. By starving yourself you can deprive your fetus or have a miscarriage – or the baby may be premature, poorly nourished with a low birthweight and birth defects.

It is normal for an expectant mother to store 3 or 4 pounds (1.5 to 2kg) of fat as a source of calories for future milk production. The storage of body fat during motherhood is one of the important basic changes in a woman, which probably evolved from our early ancestors as a means of preparing reserves for the energy needs of the newborn during lactation. Changes in metabolism and hormonal levels can make you susceptible to putting on too much weight: many obese women say their weight problems began with one or more pregnancies, so it may be that some women are sensitive to these changes. Estrogen level rises about a thousand times more than its previous blood level, although after delivery it drops sharply.

To measure for superfluous fat while pregnant, measure your upper thighs every week and keep a record of the measurement. You will be recording any increase in your own body fat as distinct from weight gain from pregnancy. Don't assume that if your baby weighs about 6 to 9 pounds (3 or 4kg) at birth, all the rest of your weight is fat. Fluid retention can account for considerable gain for some women, but after delivery you should return to normal. The American College of Obstetricians and Gynecologists considers 20 to 30 pounds (9 to 13.5kg) an acceptable range of weight increase during pregnancy, in order to deliver a healthy baby. The increase is usually made up as follows –

Baby	38 percent
Placenta	9 percent
Amniotic fluid	11 percent
Increase in weight of uterus and breasts	20 percent
Increase in weight of blood	22 percent
Total weight gain	100 percent

Normally you should have no weight increase for the first 12 weeks; an increase of about 6 pounds (3kg) during weeks 12 to 20; an increase of another 12 pounds (5.5kg) during weeks 20 to 30; a further 6 pounds (3kg) during weeks 30 to 36, and then no further weight gain for weeks 36 to 40. If you are an overweight mother, your physician may consider you should have a weight gain of perhaps only 15 pounds (7kg) so that you will have a weight loss after giving birth.

Although your body needs more fat during pregnancy, if you are eating a nutritious diet you are taking in enough fat. The increased energy requirement during pregnancy is only 15 percent additional calories − an increase of about 300 calories a day. "Eating for two" does not mean doubling your food at each meal, but choosing your calories wisely. Protein becomes more important at this time, plus carbohydrates for energy, extra iron for formation of fetal red-blood cells, calcium for bone formation, and vitamins. Regular exercise during pregnancy should be an important part of your overall fitness plan: brisk walking, golf, light weight-lifting, but not exercises with jumping movements.

6. **Breast-feeding mothers.** Up to 7 1/2 pounds (3.4kg) of body fat stored during pregnancy is used as fuel to make breast milk. This fat tends to be lost during breast feeding. You burn off 50 calories per pound of a baby's weight when you breast feed. Thus a 10-pound (4.5kg) baby costs you 500 calories a day in breast milk. So breast feeding is often recommended as a way to lose weight steadily while giving your baby important nutrients. Don't rush to diet to regain your figure, as a restriction on calories during lactation may decrease the amount of milk you produce. Aim at a slow loss of no more than 3 1/2 pounds (1.6kg) a month for the first six months. Instead of counting calories, cut the fat and sugar. Exercising after breast feeding is best, because full breasts can make physical activity uncomfortable, and fat-burning during exercise may result in more acidity of the milk.

7. **Middle age**. After about the age of 40, dietary needs are different from what they were in earlier years. Even with the same food and usual amount of exercise, you may find it easy to gain pounds probably because of a change in metabolism. For a woman, the middle years bring menopause when she ceases to menstruate. Menopause decreases the natural production of the estrogen hormone, possibly leading to an increase in the loss of calcium from bones, causing brittle-bone conditions. [See *OSTEOPOROSIS: Brittle Bones and The Calcium Crisis*, Pennant Books] Be sure to have adequate calcium as part of a balanced diet, along with daily exercise, to prevent bone-thinning, but a lean cuisine to avoid excess poundage – for instance, skim milk, lowfat yogurt and reduced-fat cheeses. Postmenopausal women have a slower and declining function in kidneys and liver, a decrease in digestive enzymes to handle large amounts of fatty foods, and when foods are not fully metabolized, they can add to fat deposits on hips, thighs and breasts.

If you are prescribed estrogens to relieve menopausal symptoms, the result may be weight gain and water retention. Because estrogens are largely responsible for the distribution of subcutaneous fat, with hormone therapy you can quickly gain inches on hips and breasts. Breasts may become tender and full as a result of fluid retention and stimulated mammary glands. Diet has to be carefully watched: reduce table salt as well as fats. At the same time, estrogen therapy may reduce the risk of heart disease in postmenopausal women by preventing a rise in blood cholesterol.

8. **Old age**. By the age of 70, your kidney and liver functions may decline by 30 to 50 percent. As you become older you need fewer calories and less fat than younger adults, but not less protein, vitamins and minerals. Gentle exercise in later years is vital, depending upon how active you can be. Many people assume that becoming overweight is simply a natural part of growing old, but it doesn't have to be accepted. It is often the natural outcome of poor food habits and too much sitting still. You can make poor choices when food shopping, if you are on a small

budget or if you have lost interest in preparing and eating food. You may be less able to smell or taste foods, or have problems with teeth or dentures. Coupled with the possible constant use of some medications, changes can occur in the nutrients needed by your body, their amounts, and how your body uses them. Nutrient deficiencies can occur in later years, although it is not known whether they may be due to poor eating or changes in the way your body absorbs nutrients. Generally speaking, there is a decrease in the percentage of metabolically-active lean tissue (including muscle) and an increase in the percentage of fat deposits. This changing ratio alters metabolism, reducing the BMR; a decline in activity reduces caloric needs still further. Whatever your age, a varied diet is the best way to get all the nutrients you need, but with a limit to fats.

Obesity can be a complicated matter, involving but not limited to:
- Cultural attitudes, the way our society views weight control.
- Physiology, with sex and genetics establishing where you deposit fat.
- Social events, with many centered around food and eating.
- Food-buying habits, determined by your built-in desire for certain tastes (sweet, salty or bitter) and textures (creamy, smooth and buttery, crunchy and crisp, or chewy).
- Religious food laws and taboos.
- The extent of your exposure to food advertising in television programs, magazines, newspapers and city billboards, that tempt you with mouth-watering pictures to buy and eat more than you need. Low-fat fruits and vegetables have a low advertising profile compared to the billion-dollar campaigns boosting fat-laden processed foods and fast foods.
- Your attitude to exercise — whether you think it fun and the natural thing to do, or a terrible bore.
- Family income, interacting with genetic factors. Lower income groups tend to be more overweight. As families climb the economic ladder, affluent men become even fatter whereas women tend to become slimmer.

- Human emotions, with overeating providing comfort in times of anger, boredom, depression due to the loss of a loved one or the loss of a job, fear, frustration, jealousy or stress. But problems are not solved by eating unwisely — obesity only creates serious problems for your health and shortens your life.

Being fat is up to you.

You have a choice: eat as you like and take your chances, or change bad eating habits and take charge of your health. A good place to start scaling down is by eating less fat with its high concentration of calories, and by resolving to make the effort to exercise more. By having a new attitude towards food, you can experience new tastes and pleasures at mealtime. Start by avoiding the greasy, the salty and the sugary-sweet that only disguise the real flavors of natural whole food as it should taste.

6

From Theory To Practice

Food, glorious food!

Food is not just a necessity, but one of life's pleasures. But subtracting the fat from food doesn't mean that you are taking away that pleasure. Gourmet cooks and chefs are redirecting their culinary skills and finding that gastronomic happiness need not depend on butter, cream and vast servings of fat-laden beef, pork and duck. Dishes can be leaner and still be appetizing, mouth-watering − even exotic − that you can present with flair and pride. Even the French have turned away from their *haute cuisine* of rich meats smothered with rich sauces and voluptuous coatings of eggs and cream, so eating well is not under threat. It is now more chic to prepare food in the leaner, lighter style of *nouvelle cuisine* that is now supplanting old methods and ingredients.

Some people crave fat more than others, and no one has said that cutting down on fat is easy. Tradition is a powerful force in determining the food you buy, eat and enjoy, and it may be hard at first to change some long-established, deep-rooted eating habits. But that doesn't mean that a target of 30 percent for fat calories is unattainable. For a start, just don't make an entire meal out of high-fat foods.

STRATEGY FOR CUTTING FAT

✓ Take an overall view of the type of meals and snacks you generally eat, and count the grams of fat. Home-prepared foods put *you* in control.

✓ Shopping: Go for skim milk, nonfat dairy products, well-trimmed lean meat, and fewer processed foods.

✓ Be a label reader.

✓ Review recipes and cooking methods.

✓ Review kitchen equipment.

✓ Use caution when dining out.

✓ Be selective of fast foods.

AN OVERALL VIEW

Shop right, cook right, eat right, live right.

Where are you and where do you want to be in terms of your own state of health? What sort of eater are you? Keep a brief diary to jot down when you eat and what you eat − and drink − snacks, nibbles and extras as well as main meals. Note what was in that food and check the fat content of each item (see Appendix III). Or use your personal computer to determine the saturates you eat, with a nutrient analysis program such as the DINE system (from DINE Systems, Inc., 724 Robin Road, West Amherst, New York 14228). Don't think of "dieting" as such; you are modifying your eating patterns. Where do you need to make changes? Reverse bad habits? Balance your diet to maintain a variety of foods?

Determine your personal caloric needs, from which you estimate your daily quota of fat calories, as detailed in Table 6 on page 101. For example, a man needing 2400 calories should limit fat calories to 720, or 80 grams of fat, for a goal of 30 percent; a woman needing 1600 calories should limit fat calories to 480, or 53 grams of fat.

How much total fat are you presently eating? Fat is fat, whether you are eating butter, margarine, olive oil or saturated animal fat. You've got to cut fat across the board. Rather than counting every single gram of fat in your favorite foods, you may find it easier to identify and cut back on the major sources of fat in your daily meals. And rather than give up one of your favorite foods entirely, simply eat a smaller amount, have it less often, or see if it is available in a reduced-fat style.

Turn back to Table 1 on page 22 that gives the percentage of fat in common foods. How does your usual shopping list compare with these groups? You can do considerable fat-cutting by keeping to foods on the left-hand page. The more items you can choose from the left side and fewer foods from the right, the less fat you will be eating.

High-fat extra foods such as gravies, sauces, pies, French fries, potato chips, salad dressings and bread spreads should be the first to cut from your list. Sausages, cured meats, bacon, ham, lard, sour cream, double cream, whole milk and whole-milk products are high-fat, high-cholesterol culprits; reduced-fat alternatives are often available. Be aware that some foods can be high in fat but low in cholesterol (for instance, vegetable oil), others high in cholesterol but low in fat (for instance, eggs).

Choose and use these foods:
- All vegetables and fruits, except coconut; fruit and vegetable juices.
- Pasta, rice, potatoes, oatmeal, wheat bran, oat bran and other cold cereals, hot cereals, wholegrain bread, English muffins, soda crackers.
- Skim milk, nonfat yogurt, lowfat cottage cheese, lowfat ricotta.
- Egg whites.
- Clear soups and broths.
- Lean cuts of beef, lamb, pork or veal (fat trimmed off); skinless chicken and turkey; fish, clams, mussels, shrimp, lobster.
- Fruit sherbets, sorbets, ice milk, frozen yogurt, frozen fruit bars; angel-food cake, jams and jellies, gelatin desserts; unbuttered popcorn, chestnuts; peanut butter in moderation.
- Black coffee and tea, in moderation.
- Wine, beer and liquors in moderation.

Limit or eliminate these foods:
- Butter, margarine or shortening made from saturated fats, lard and bacon fat, mayonnaise, salad dressing, saturated oils, palm oil, coconut oil and coconut milk.
- Whole milk, cream, sour cream, cream sauces and soups, custard-style yogurt, custard, gravies, hard and soft cheese including cream cheese.
- Whole eggs and egg yolks.
- French fries and other fried foods.
- Hamburgers, sausages, salami, bacon and hot dogs; fatty cuts of beef, lamb or pork; organ meats, goose, duck, and poultry skin; caviar and fish roe.
- Pastry, doughnuts, and butter cookies; ice cream, milk shakes and frozen tofu; chocolate and caramels.

When you remove fat from meals, what do you replace it with? Complex carbohydrates such as wholewheat breads, grains and pastas, plus fresh fruits and vegetables. Forget the myth that carbs are fattening. Simple carbs such as sugar and soft drinks you can leave on the supermarket shelf, but complex carbs fill you up with only half the caloric cost of fats. A potato doesn't make you fat, a slice of wholegrain bread doesn't – but the butter you put on it does!

Assess your meals for each day or for the week. You may find it helpful to develop meal plans for the whole week to make shopping easier. Then stock up on a variety of lowfat foods, filling your refrigerator with fresh produce and your pantry with whole grains and spices. (Don't use the term "larder.") What is in the kitchen and what you eat every day is what really counts. Having a super-rich decadent dessert *occasionally* won't hurt – and may be good for the soul! If you're dining out, and a rich gourmet meal is unavoidable, or if you have to have fast food on the run, strike a balance by cutting out fat at other meals on that day. Blood cholesterol levels and waistline measurements don't respond to a single day's food intake. They reflect the sum of the fats you have eaten over the past several weeks.

SHOPPING

Dairy Produce. Since whole milk is a high-fat food, start cutting fat by buying the right kind of milk. Don't cut down on drinking milk as you need its calcium to make and maintain strong bones – unless you should avoid dairy products for other medical reasons. What you don't need is the fat to clog your bloodstream or store around your middle.

As milk is on nearly everyone's shopping list, let's clear up any confusion about its fat content:

An 8oz. cup of nonfat skim milk has 0 grams of fat (no fat calories) out of a total 85 calories:

0 percent of the calories are from fat.

An 8oz. cup of lowfat milk (2 percent fat by weight) has 5g of fat (45 calories), out of a total 120 calories:

37 percent of the calories are from fat.

An 8oz. cup of whole milk (3.3 percent fat by weight) has 8g of fat (72 calories), out of a total 150 calories:

48 percent of the calories are from fat.

Go for nonfat and let the dairy industry worry about what to do with the fat. (But it is unwise to give young babies nonfat milk unless under doctor's orders.) Skim milk is heart-healthy, with the good nutrients of whole milk but minus the extra calories and unwanted fat, although when fat is removed, there is some loss of vitamins A and D. Avoid goats milk, condensed milk and evaporated whole milk as these are all high-fat. Shun imitation or substitute milk in which butterfat has been replaced with vegetable oil; the oil most commonly used is coconut, which is more saturated than butterfat. Many imitation milks also have a higher sodium content than real milk.

Most of us think of cheese as healthful, but you may not be doing your health a favor by replacing meat with cheese. From a fat and nutrient standpoint you are better off with lean meat. Most cheeses are good sources of quality protein, but the protein comes at a price: high fat and thus high calorie. Generally, fresh cheeses contain less fat and are less caloric than aged cheeses. Limit servings to one ounce or less, eating it with other foods that are low in fat.

Next time at the supermarket, make a note to buy lowfat spreads for breads, lowfat dairy products and reduced-fat cheeses. Don't be misled by artificial creams and imitation sour creams that are often synthesized from tropical oils which have just as much fat as real cream.

Meats and Meat Products. If you eat meat, keep portions small. Exactly how much fat do red meats contain? The amounts vary, depending on how the animal was bred and raised, the location of the meat cut, the amount of marbling and the amount of trimming. Farmers are breeding leaner animals and raising them on more nutritious feed. Lean (Lite) Beef has been introduced, emphasizing reduced fat, and hogs which were formerly raised to provide large amounts of lard now have more lean protein.

The Department of Agriculture grades beef "Prime," "Choice," and "Select," with the main indicator for grading being the amount of marbling – the streaks of fat that interlace lean muscle tissue. So the fattier the cut, the more expensive it is – and the less healthy it is. *The fat content varies more from cut to cut than it does from grade to grade.* Choose the leanest cuts you can find and afford, looking for packages with as little marbling as possible, with little visible fat. The "trim" on a piece of meat is the fat around the edge, which should be no more than 1/4 inch. You yourself can make many cuts leaner by trimming off even more fat.

For years, fat in meat was assumed to be synonymous with flavor and tenderness, but with sensible cooking methods you can decrease fat without having a family revolt. Look for eye of round, top round, bottom round, round tip roast, tenderloin, veal cutlets, leg of lamb and lean ground beef or ground turkey. Ground meat can look quite red but still b · .atty; ground turkey may include turkey skin. The best way to be sure of what you're getting is to buy the meat or poultry and grind it yourself. Don't keep chicken and turkey just for holidays or fish just for Fridays. Replace red meats with fish two or three times a week.

Made-up meat products such as frozen pies, cold cuts, links and brown-and-serve sausages can be minefields because most have too much fat and it is concealed. If you cannot avoid them, use them sparingly. What goes in a sausage? Before you buy, check the label or ask the butcher for details. Lower-fat sausages are available with about half the usual fat — they may be higher priced, but worth the extra cost in terms of good health.

Processed foods. Develop a preference for foods as close as possible to their natural state. While many people are eating less visible fat, they simultaneously have increased their consumption of *invisible* fats in ready-prepared foods. During the past twenty years, there has been a steady increase of fat in U.S. food supplies, with the increase due almost entirely to vegetable fats including the highly saturated tropical oils.

You can take it for granted that most snack and processed foods are loaded with dangerous fat. By removing ready-prepared foods from your shopping list, you can subtract significant amounts of calorie-laden fats from your diet, as well as sugar, salt and many dubious chemicals. Many have hidden fats or oils when you least expect them. Stop buying them, and the manufacturers will stop producing them.

Years ago, good food could be defined generally as hot, homemade and wholesome, with seasonal natural ingredients that were no mystery. Today's "good foods" are enriched, fortified, pre-salted, pre-sweetened, quick to heat, quick to eat, good "keepers," prettily wrapped to conceal ingredients known only by chemists in the food industry. And the food chemists work to cost guidelines created by accountants, to produce items as cheaply as possible and maximize profits for the manufacturers. The technology of food manufacturing, processing and preservation has undergone a revolution in the past thirty years, and a fiercely competitive battle among food firms is waged in supermarkets to obtain preferred shelf space. Consequently, shoppers are confronted by a bewildering array of choices and an avalanche of new food items — frozen, freeze-dried, dehydrated, vacuum-sealed, concentrated and irradiated. Even the most conscientious shopper can be confused in the supermarket by the displays of bright colorful boxes, and beguiled by TV ads devoted to glorifying the fattiest foods. Your major concerns when shopping are: 1) taste, 2) ease of preparation and 3) economy.

You are probably eating a greater variety of foods than ever before, but how healthy are some of these new products? Do you know exactly what you are eating? Food additives have apparently become indispensable to food production and marketing – chemicals that prevent spoilage, enhance taste, create texture and keep ingredients in suspension. Many of them are derived from fats and oils.

LABELING

Some processed foods are more harmful than others, making it vital for you to be a label reader.

Take a look at a few popular terms that are used on labels of processed foods, to see the misleading marketing and the obvious or not-so-obvious deceptions:

"All natural." The use of the words is not regulated and to many people it means "safe," but the phrase simply means the package has ingredients derived from natural sources – the food may still contain excessive amounts of "all natural" fats, refined sugar and salt.

"All-vegetable" or "100% vegetable" means that no animal fat has been used. Frequently, though, foods such as shortening may be more saturated with tropical oils, or oils that have undergone hydrogenation.

"Enriched." You may think you are buying a superior product with something extra here, but being enriched means nutrients removed in processing have been added back. If the product has been "enriched" by pumping in fat, who needs it?

"Fiber" is popular on labels – but which kind of fiber are you buying? Pectins? Gums? The bran naturally present in whole-grain cereals? Fiber from soy bran, corn bran or wood cellulose that is put in some baked goods? No one knows the long-term effects of wood consumption on the human body, or whether these fibers behave similarly to whole wheat in the gastro-intestinal tract.

"Fortified." A squirt of synthetic vitamins and minerals may be all you are buying. Processors don't fortify foods to deliver nutrients to the customer – they fortify them so that they can label them as fortified which sells the products. Fortification doesn't redeem foods if they contain excessive amounts of fat, sugar, salt or dubious additives.

"Instant." Each time a food undergoes further processing, more nutrients are lost and some undesirable elements may be added, so you end up with various combinations of emulsifiers, preservatives, stabilizers and artificial flavoring frequently derived from fat sources.

"Light" or "Lite" foods may or may not have fewer calories. When it comes to food, a consistent definition of the word does not exist. Light on a package of cheese means one thing; on a bag of potato chips it means something else. Light beer may have fewer calories or be a term referring to color.

"Low calorie." Frozen diet meals often keep their promise of a reduced number of calories, but many are too high in fat and salt, or contain dubious chemicals and additives.

"No cholesterol." Be wary. Such products, although containing no cholesterol, may still have large quantities of fat. Examples of no-cholesterol but high-fat foods are peanut butters and all vegetable oils. Powdered nondairy creamers have no cholesterol, but are high in palm-, palm-kernel or coconut oil, with saturates that tend to raise serum cholesterol.

"Nutritious." Sounds good, doesn't it, but what does it really mean? It doesn't stand for any specific food value. In other words, on a food label it is worthless.

Ignore the popular terms splashed in bold type across packaging. Take a moment to read carefully the nutrition information label, and the detailed list of ingredients, to see for yourself how much fat you are buying. Only in this way can you make informed decisions as to whether you really need or should avoid processed foods containing large amounts of grease, oil or fat. Nutrition information is usually an analysis of the product performed by the manufacturer, or a calculation based on actual or typical values of the ingredients used. Food manufacturers follow a standard format.

The real problem today is that information on labels is incomplete and inadequate. They give serving size, servings per package, and details of nutrition in each serving, but first ask yourself if the serving size on the label is the same amount that *you* would use. Then food labels can be misleading because they list fat by weight, whereas nutritionists look at the percentage of fat out of total calories, which can be a much higher figure, because a gram of fat has twice the calories of protein and carbohydrate. For instance, some lunch meats can be labeled 97 percent fat-free by weight, but the percentage of total calories that come from fat can still be high. To determine the fat percentage, multiply the grams of fat by 9, and divide by the total calories.

And it is crucial to know how much is saturated fat, since *blood cholesterol levels are raised more by fat saturates than by the cholesterol you eat.* When a label says a product contains "one or more of the following oils" and the list includes tropical oils along with, for instance, safflower or corn oil, making no distinction about their saturation, the consumer is confused and uncertain about the health risk. What is actually inside the package is anybody's guess. Rather than take a gamble, pick another brand or another product.

Go for the products bearing labels specifying that the contents have reduced fat:

"Extra lean" when contents must contain 5 percent or less fat, and the actual amount must be shown on the label.

"Lean" and "lowfat" when the products must contain 10 percent or less fat.

"Leaner" and "lower fat" when the food must contain 25 percent less fat than other similar products.

"Lite" can have various meanings and may refer to less fat, fewer calories, less sodium or lighter color.

Only a few product labels give information on cholesterol content, but if you want specific details, the manufacturers are usually able to supply them when you write to the address on the product label.

Future foods

When is a fat not a fat? In the next few years you will see ingredient labels listing "engineered" compounds such as *N-Oil*, *polydextrose* and *sucrose polyester* being used to replace up to half the amount of regular fat in everyday foods. These chemicals have been created to simulate the smoothness and richness we associate with fat, mimicking the texture of fat particles and thus fooling our taste buds, but at the same time reducing calories and cholesterol. Artificial fat substitutes fall into three general categories:

emulsified starches - mixtures of starch and water, used in some salad dressings;

emulsified proteins – gelatin/water mixtures now being test-marketed in butter and margarine, products that can be used in baking and light frying. Another version, under the brand name "Simplesse," based on milk and egg proteins, cannot be cooked since heat causes it to gel. Simplesse contains 1.3 calories per gram compared to fat's 9 calories per gram. You may find it used in ice cream, cheese spreads, dips, margarine, mayonnaise and salad dressings;

synthetic chemicals – such as sucrose polyester, synthesized from edible oils bonded to sucrose (table sugar). Sucrose polyester (SPE), sometimes referred to as olestra, may be used for deep frying and in cooked and uncooked foods, such as cooking oils and shortenings, potato chips, low-calorie cookies and ice cream. Although sounding more like material for making sportswear that doesn't need ironing, sucrose polyester looks and tastes like a vegetable oil, and acts like normal fat during cooking, but provides no calories. The fat molecules are too large for the digestive enzyme lipase to break down, so they pass through the body without being absorbed into the bloodstream.

Some of these compounds still have to undergo government evaluation and approval, and even then, doubts remain about their complete safety. The Center for Science in the Public Interest, the consumer group based in Washington, D.C., has suggested that olestra causes leukemia, tumors, liver damage and birth defects in laboratory rats. So, even when these questions are resolved, it remains a personal decision: do you want to buy foods containing these additives? It is not just fat, cholesterol and calories in food that you should be concerned about, but the nutritive value and intrinsic wholesomeness.

REVIEW RECIPES AND COOKING METHODS
The food you buy is only part of the story about cutting fat. The way you prepare and serve food can be just as important. As a general rule you should be doing less frying, barbecuing and smoking of foods, and choosing more often −

✓ Raw
✓ Baking
✓ Boiling
✓ Braising
✓ Frying in nonstick cookware, using no fat or oil
✓ Frying using only nonstick cooking sprays
        (which contain a trace of oil)
✓ Grilling, with no added fat, and flame above food
✓ Microwave cooking
✓ Poaching
✓ Pressure-cooking
✓ Roasting
✓ Simmering
✓ Slow cooking in a crockpot
✓ Steaming
✓ Stewing
✓ Stir-frying in a tiny amount of oil

Part of the joy of cooking is the inclusion of special recipes, particularly those handed down through families, but unfortunately many "heirloom treasures" are loaded with fat and calories or use unsuitable old-fashioned greasy methods. You may find recipes suitable for today's lean cuisine among cookbooks of the Spartan 1940s when butter, eggs and meat were in short supply and used sparingly. You need to bring them up to date. Take a few minutes to go through your favorites and study them critically. You can modify many recipes, making notes where fat can be reduced or eliminated entirely, without changing the character of the dish, with little if any compromise on flavor, texture, or finished appearance. Often the effect on a dish is small, whereas nutritionally the difference can be great. All it takes is some common sense in experimenting and switching quantities, and a bit of psychology in steering your family towards healthier eating. The chart below shows the calories from fat in recipe measures:

8 oz of oil = 1 cup = 16 Tbsp = 48 tsp = about 2000 calories
4 oz of oil = 1/2 cup = 8 Tbsp = 24 tsp = about 1000 calories
2 oz of oil = 1/4 cup = 4 Tbsp = 12 tsp = about 500 calories
1 oz of oil = 1/8 cup = 2 Tbsp = 6 tsp = about 250 calories
1/2 oz of oil = 1 Tbsp = 3 tsp = about 125 calories
1 tsp of oil = about 42 calories

Watch out for fats and oils that can be 1) a food ingredient, 2) coated with them, 3) cooked with them, or 4) added at serving time. Here are some practical suggestions –

- Decrease fat or eliminate it entirely in marinades. Soak food in acidic liquids such as lime juice, wine or vinegar to soften muscle fibers and add extra flavor.
- Go ethnic: almost every country has dishes that combine plenty of rice, pasta and vegetables, with little or no meat. Try skewered kabobs, alternating cubes of meat and vegetables. You may like to take a cooking class in Chinese stir-fry, Japanese sushi, or pasta-making.
- With Chinese-style stir-frying, use the tiniest amount of hot oil and finely-chopped foods sliced against the grain to tenderize tough cuts. Make tough meat more tender by pounding and cutting into thin strips before cooking. Make sure cooking oil is sufficiently hot before adding food, to avoid fat being absorbed.

- Poach food, instead of frying, using a nonfat liquid such as chicken broth or tomato juice to prepare vegetables, or Worcestershire sauce to sauté mushrooms.
- Try switching highly-saturated fats such as butter, lard and shortening to soft tub margarine or PUFA vegetable oils, and try reducing the amount. As a general rule, substituting oil for shortening can be tricky unless specified in recipes. Low-calorie fats or diet margarine can be a help, but usually they shouldn't be heated as they lose the water and air incorporated into their composition.
- For butter flavor minus the calories, try commercial butter-flavored seasonings.
- If you like the flavor of bacon fat, chicken fat or lard with certain foods, you may have to toss out the recipe or sacrifice that taste.
- Blend lean ground meat with cooked rice to "stretch" it and further reduce fat.
- Before adding meatballs to a sauce, oven-bake them on a rack, in a standard oven or microwave. The excess fat from the meat should drain off into the pan below and not into your sauce.
- When you roast meat, make sure it is placed well above drippings. Discard drippings – don't be tempted to use them in frying or cooking other dishes.
- Meats should not be floured or breaded before browning or roasting because the coating acts like a sponge and absorbs the meat fats.
- If your family insists on gravy, first drain off fat, and make a sauce with the sediment and clear broth. For chicken gravy without chicken fat, use clear skimmed chicken broth and PUFA margarine.
- After cooking soups, stews, broths, gravies and sauces, use an ice cube to pick up any floating fat. Or chill overnight to harden fat for easy removal before reheating and serving.
- Before serving foods, blot surface fats with paper towel.
- Cut back on recipes using whipped cream and cream sauces, rich gravies, dishes with Strogonoff or au gratin in the name,

Hollandaise sauce, cream cheese, sour cream, bottled dressings and crumbled bacon (real or synthetic).
- Consider how eggs are used in recipes: are they for binding, for browning, or to help the dish to rise? Can you omit them? You can often reduce the number of eggs needed for a recipe, substituting a tablespoon of water for each egg you omit. Or use egg whites without the yolks (2 egg whites = 1 whole egg).
- Try egg-substitutes. Although usually high in sodium content, they are lower in cholesterol.
- Salt may be omitted or reduced in many recipes. You need no salt when boiling potatoes, vegetables, rice, pasta and so on. Season with zesty herbs, spices or lemon juice. Use a salt-substitute only if you must, and use sparingly to avoid any possible bitter taste.
- You may be able to reduce the sugar content in a recipe by using a sugar-substitute, although, as a general rule, a non-caloric sugar-substitute cannot be used in a cake. Try adding more spices and dried fruit to recipes instead of sugar.

REVIEW KITCHEN EQUIPMENT

Old pans may be poor conductors of heat. If you are doing a quick stir-fry, the oil may not become sufficiently hot and may start soaking into food before you have finished cooking. Using some of your pans out of sentiment because they were wedding presents, or given to you by your mother, makes no sense when trying to cut fat and calories; retire them to the back of the cupboard. Cast a critical eye on utensils, cooking pans and equipment to see if they measure up as fat cutters:

A *blender* can turn vegetables (fresh or leftovers), broth and cooked potatoes into voluptuous "cream" soups. A quick spin can produce lowfat homemade mayonnaise or dressings superior to commercial brands. You can make milk shakes with powdered skim milk, diet lemonade and ice cubes; for mock sour cream, blend cottage cheese with a teaspoon of milk and a teaspoon of lemon juice.

The *broiler* should be used whenever possible (instead of frying pan) with no added fat, allowing any drippings to accumulate below and be discarded.

Casseroles use cheaper cuts of meat in smaller quantities, combined with lots of vegetables. Before adding meat or chicken to the dish, remove all visible fat and skin, and spoon off all fat that rises to the top at the end of cooking.

Dishes. Use smaller salad plates for entrees, to help you with portion control if you are watching calories.

Fat separator. A simple jug with a low spout, handy for quick separation of fats that rise to the top of gravies, stock, soups and sauces.

Measuring spoons help you add the precise amount of oil to a pan or bowl instead of guessing and pouring it straight in.

Microwave oven. Fat called for in recipes can be greatly reduced when microwaving because the moist method of cooking retains flavor and prevents food from sticking to pans, with no add-itional oils necessary for greasing.

Nonstick cooking sprays. These are usually liquid lecithin derived from soybeans. A spray of about 5 seconds will put about 1 gram of fat into your pan or baking dish. This can be a considerable saving compared to a chunk of fat or spoonful of oil.

Nonstick pans have a chemical coating on the surface where contact with food is made, the basic underlying pan usually being aluminum. One or two brands of nonstick pans have recessed dimples on the cooking surface that not only ensure no sticking but catch any fat that drips from food while cooking. These pans can be a boon for a lean cuisine if you take care not to scratch the nonstick surface.

Poachers. Small ones for eggs, large ones for whole fish.

Pressure-cookers. There has been a rebirth in the popularity of these old-time cookers because of their ability to tenderize tough cuts of meat and vegetables in stews, flavorful stocks and pots of beans. They are timesavers in busy households, while saving two-thirds the amount of gas or electricity. Several brands have bright new designs to make these cookers safe, quiet, and of durable construction.

A *rack* will keep roasts from sitting in drippings while cooking.

Sauté pan. Instead of oil or fat, use a little liquid such as broth or water. Or use a nonstick cooking spray, or wipe liquid lecithin on pan surface with paper towel.

Sharp knives are necessary for trimming all visible fat, and removing bones to reach hidden fat pockets.

A *slotted spoon* will lift meat out of drippings after browning.

Slow cookers. The slow-cooking process tenderizes cheap but tough meat cuts or a potful of simmering beans and other vegetables. Some have browning elements; some don't.

Use a *steamer* for cooking fish and vegetables lightly, to preserve the most vitamins, minerals and other nutrients, using no fat.

Wok or *karhai.* If you must fry, make it a quick stir-fry using a steep-sided, round-bottomed pan such as a wok (East Indians call it a karhai), using only a small amount of oil — a teaspoon or two is often enough. Food has less time to absorb the fat. Choose one with a nonstick surface; a dome lid is helpful for fast steaming vegetables. Use a PUFA cooking oil (safflower, sunflower, soybean or corn) because they reach high temperatures without smoking excessively, or a monounsaturated olive oil to contribute flavor. Three basic rules: 1) chop all ingredients into small pieces or thin strips across the grain, 2) use high heat for fast cooking, and 3) stir frequently and serve promptly.

DINING OUT

Eating at home is usually more healthful and certainly less expensive than dining out, but most of us look forward to going to a restaurant once in a while to meet friends, discuss business, try new foods, or simply have a change of routine and get out of the house. But break the correlation of going out to eat and *over*eating.

When you know you are eating out, have nonfat or lowfat, low-salt foods such as fresh fruits and raw vegetables for other meals and snacks that day. Give yourself healthy carbohydrates and fiber to counterbalance the restaurant fats you may be unable to avoid, and to keep your total dietary fats on target for that day.

You can avoid eating a lot of fat or excessive calories by knowing some of the pitfalls, being aware of what you are ordering, and making sure you are served exactly what you ordered. Don't be afraid to tell the waiter you don't want your food cooked with butter, salt or monosodium glutamate (MSG). Ask the waiter if he can recommend a lowfat menu item – but don't take his word for it. Don't be self-conscious about asking what the ingredients of a dish are, and how it is prepared. Generally, the better restaurants have grown accustomed to special requests, and are usually able to serve lighter, lowfat meals. Order à la carte rather than complete dinners. If the menu seems hopelessly overloaded with fatty items, ask for a heap of freshly-steamed vegetables or a double order of a salad.

Appetizers can be a fresh fruit cup, fruit juice, melon slice or half grapefruit. Consommés and clear soups are best as they generally have little fat. Order foods broiled, baked, steamed or boiled. Keep away from foods fried in fat or prepared with cream sauces. Foods that are breaded before frying are particularly bad because the coating soaks up fat like a sponge. If menu items include sauces, gravies and salad dressings, ask for them to be served on the side, then *you* can decide what to have.

Have the rolls removed from the table if you think you can't resist slathering them with butter while waiting for your main course. If you are hungry, ask for your salad to be served immediately. Fill up on vegetables first, or other foods that are usually low in fat and calories. A baked potato or plain rice is usually an excellent choice. Keep meat to a minimum, and order it cooked medium to well – the longer meat cooks, the more fat is rendered from it. Be aware that steakhouse toppings such as onions, mushrooms or green peppers are usually sautéed in butter. Do you need them?

Portion control is a good way to avoid calories you don't need. Become an expert on estimating portion sizes: the size of an average woman's palm is about 3 inches square by 3/4 inch thick (7.5cm square by 2cm thick); a portion of meat approximately that size weighs 3 ounces (85g). If servings are over-generous, leave some on your plate – you don't have to belong to the "clean plate club" and finish everything just because you are paying for it. Alternatively, you can share the meal with your table companion, or take the food home so none is wasted.

Ethnic food and foreign cuisine is trendy, and trying new food flavors is always interesting. Each kind of ethnic cuisine has benefits as well as drawbacks. In French restaurants, look for lighter style items on the menu, in the manner of *nouvelle cuisine*. Good selections would be foods simply broiled without butter, or dishes cooked in wine, rather than prepared with cream and butter sauces. Chinese restaurants can be good because their usual custom is to serve mounds of vegetables and small amounts of meat, but avoid the salty sauces − soy, oyster or black-bean. Ask the waiter which type of oil is used in the kitchen and if MSG is added during food preparation. Choose quick stir-fry dishes and plain boiled rice, avoiding deep-fried foods and fried rice. Indian, Indonesian and Thai restaurants may use ghee (see Appendix I), coconut oil or coconut milk − all high in saturates and to be avoided. It's fun to go to Japanese sushi (raw fish) bars occasionally, or restaurants featuring teppanyaki where foods are quickly and lightly sautéed. The pitfalls in Italian restaurants can be entrées that are deep-fried, with thick batter coatings, or prepared with high-fat cheeses. Pasta topped with a marinara sauce, a meatless tomato sauce, vegetable or seafood sauce is an appropriate choice. Order chicken cacciatore cooked in tomato sauce instead of chicken Parmesan with its breading and cheese; or you may prefer veal piccata lightly sautéed with lemon. Breadsticks, without butter of course, make for good crunching while you are waiting to be served. Mexican restaurants are becoming popular worldwide. Avoid crisp corn tortillas (which are fried) and choose soft flour tortillas (which are baked or microwaved). Try *seviche* − marinated raw fish. Instead of lard-laden refried beans, order Mexican rice. Refuse extra cheese, sour cream and guacamole (avocado dip).

You don't have to ignore the dessert menu, but do say a firm "No thanks" to the chef's rich cakes and pies, cheesecakes, tortes and other glories topped or sandwiched with whipped (real or artificial) cream! You don't need them clogging your bloodstream. Desserts can be chilled wedges of melon, pieces of fresh fruit, a bowl of luscious berries, fruit salad, stewed fruit, fruit sherbet or, occasionally, ice cream. Ask if the restaurant can serve ice milk or frozen yogurt. Maybe you fancied something from the cheeseboard? Most cheeses are high-fat and usually high-sodium, especially Camembert, hard Cheddar and Stilton. Dutch Edam or some soft cheese spreads may have less fat than other varieties (see Appendix III). Ask for reduced-fat cheeses. Keep the portion very small: one ounce or less. Thin Melba toast, crispbreads, flatbreads or unsalted wheat crackers would be the best choices for this course. If you must have "butter," make it a thin smear of a PUFA diet margarine or lowfat spread.

What are you having to drink? Choose skim milk, decaffeinated coffee without cream, herbal teas, mineral waters with a twist of lemon. If you have alcoholic drinks, take them in moderation: a glass or two of wine, champagne or sherry. Say no to spirits and mixed cocktails that can be highly alcoholic and caloric; drinks made with cream or milk, eggnogs, flips and cream liqueurs are obviously high-fat as well.

Don't go hog-wild at parties! Entertaining in your home is generally easier than in someone else's, because you can control recipes and the dishes you serve your guests. But when you are the guest and not the host, mention that you are fighting fat. Ask friends and family to help you keep your resolve to reduce fat calories. Learn to be assertive in a pleasant graceful manner. Don't feel that because you refuse an offer of unsuitable food, you are personally rejecting your hostess. Have a low-cal, lowfat snack before leaving home to avoid arriving at a party over-hungry.

Buffet parties with unlimited amounts of food are a temptation to overeat. Plan beforehand to eat only a specific amount and *not* overdo it, trying to avoid dishes with excessive amounts of fat or rich sauces and dressings. Don't let someone else bring you a plate already piled high with buffet food or a bowl filled with snacks you know you shouldn't eat. Holidays can be a particularly difficult time, when you are confronted with groaning tables of delicious-looking foods, many of which are probably not compatible with a lowfat, low-cholesterol regimen. But when planning festive meals, traditional holiday food can still be fun if you give careful thought to modifying your recipes to keep them low in fat and to control portions. Serve dishes with attractive decorations and garnishes to give them extra eye-appeal.

Summertime barbecues can still sizzle occasionally. Spray the grates with nonstick vegetable coating and grill skinned chicken, turkey or fish, and potatoes or corn wrapped in foil. Experiment with lemon juice and spices rather than high-sodium, high-sugar barbecue sauces. Cool watermelon, cantaloupe, fresh pineapple, and other fruits are always perfect for hot summer days.

Before you take a vacation, think back to past holidays. Did you gain weight? A cruise is bad news if its main attraction is eating. If your tour includes prepaid hotel meals or if all meals are in restaurants, you lose some control over food content. But don't feel overwhelmed – use caution when ordering food, remember portion-control, and try to do more walking or swimming. Buy fruit for lowfat snacking if you need extra nibbles. Remember that food is only one component of a holiday – a vacation can be a fun event filled with enjoying new sights and making new friendships.

Flying? Ask your travel agent or the airline to order you a lowfat, low-cholesterol meal; ask for simply-broiled fish, chicken or a vegetarian plate; scrape off sauces. When sandwiches arrive with sliced meat and cheese, remove one or other to reduce fat. Remove egg and cheese from a salad and use minimal dressing. Bypass the salt packets. Take your own fresh fruit for a snack, to avoid the inevitable salted nuts.

IN THE FAST LANE
You lead a busy life. Fast food is quick and easy. It satisfies your gnawing appetite whether at work, on the road, on vacation, or when too busy at home. Everyone's on the run and can't be bothered to cook. We expect convenience food to fill the

stomach in five minutes. The kids choose it every time. For the hurried, worried and overworked, it's pay your money, gulp it down, and hope for the best. But is it healthy? What is in it? Since fast foods and quick take-aways have become such an integral part of life, if you want to stay healthy it's crucial to use all the meal-planning techniques that you do at home.

The growth of the fast-food industry is probably due to several factors — an increase in the number of working women, more people living alone with no motivation to cook for themselves, greater informality in lifestyles, convenience while driving, and the powerful influence of advertising on TV, radio, newspapers, magazines and billboards. It is estimated that every *second* of the day, 200 people in the U.S. are ordering fast-food hamburgers — or 6.7 billion beef patties a year, worth more than $10 billion. More than 5 billion pounds of potatoes produced in the U.S. are turned into French fries for the fast-food industry. Vending machines are even popping out cups of freshly made sizzling French fries in 30 seconds. In fact, half the potatoes grown in America are made into French fries, potato chips or frozen products.

A well-balanced diet is not compromised by an occasional fast-track meal. But if you eat on the run regularly, you need to choose carefully, and try to limit how often you have this type of food.

Because most fast foods are of animal origin and most menu items are fried, the average fat content ranges between 40 and 50 percent of calories. The fat is predominantly saturated, and the high temperatures used in frying foods increase the saturation of frying oils or fats. Some outlets offer food items so fat-laden, you can almost feel your arteries stiffen as you read the menu. Fries cooked in animal fat or tropical oils can be guaranteed to raise your blood cholesterol, and the salt will cause your blood pressure to ascend to new heights. Most fast-food chains take basically good food and turn it into bad. The minute you plunge food into a fryer of hot grease, you add fat and calories. If you start with hamburgers, which have fat as they are, then put on cheese, adding still more fat, with double burgers, double cheeseburgers, and sauces based on mayonnaise, you could have over 65 grams of fat in just one meal. More than your entire day's "allowance" of fat.

You may want to avoid red meat, full of saturated fat, and choose less-fatty chicken or fish, but eating chicken or fish in a fast-food restaurant is almost as bad as eating beef. The favorable fatty-acid content in chicken and fish is destroyed by the cooking process. A Harvard Medical School analysis has shown that the fatty-acid profiles of chicken nuggets, chicken sandwiches and fish fillets resemble beef more than chicken or fish. According to industry figures, one chicken sandwich contains 42 grams of fat, equivalent to the fat content in 1 1/2 pints of rich ice cream. Chicken nuggets may be injected with ground chicken skin.

Food items are usually fried in beef tallow. Tallow is fat trimmed from meat cuts and rendered to make highly-saturated shortening. Although vegetable oil is sometimes mixed in, beef tallow is usually the main cooking oil − more saturated than lard. The reasons are simply that tallow is relatively inexpensive, it doesn't break down at higher temperatures as unsaturated vegetable oils do, and the fat is more flavorful. The largest fast-food chains make no secret about the use of beef and vegetable shortening for French fries, claiming that it produces a high quality product with a flavor customers want and are going to buy. But their use of beef tallow directly undermines the efforts of health experts trying to turn the public towards PUFA oils.

Other outlets use palm oil or coconut oil for frying − perhaps believing, mistakenly, that they are using healthful vegetable products when in fact these oils are more saturated than beef tallow. One of the large chains for fast Mexican food has been using coconut oil to fry tortillas for a variety of dishes. Movie theaters use tropical oils on popcorn.

Fast-food restaurants can be a dietary obstacle course, because much of the food is too high in terms of animal fat content, but fast chains do provide inexpensive nutritious food, and a little nutrition knowledge goes a long way in helping to make healthful menu decisions.

Does the fast-food outlet have ingredients listed with their food packaging, or is there a notice or booklet supplying nutrient content in the restaurant? Appendix IV gives some information on the nutrient content of food from some of the major chains. Use it as only a general guideline because of frequent changes in recipes, additions to menus and variations in the availability of ingredients in some areas.

Salad bars are becoming increasingly common in popular chains, primarily because consumers have wanted healthier fare. They can offer good lowfat alternatives, provided you limit spoonfuls of high-fat dressings, and toppings of crumbled fried bacon, shredded cheese, seeds, croutons and hard-boiled eggs.

In pizzerias, thin-crust pizza is not bad, if you go easy on the cheese, and avoid toppings such as pepperoni, sausages, olives, or salty anchovies packed in oil, which can multiply fat calories. Add extra tomatoes, onions, green peppers and mushrooms.

Take a look at a fast menu and check the possibilities for choosing healthier alternatives.

Refuse:	**Choose:**
Hamburgers, cheeseburgers	Salad bars, fish or chicken (strip the skin and batter).
Deluxe, whopper, double-decker, super, extra crispy	Smallest version with fewer calories and fatty sauces.
Hot dogs and frankfurters	Plain roast beef, barbecued beef.
White buns	Wholewheat or multigrain buns.
Breaded, battered, fried	Baked or grilled.
Mayonnaise	Low-calorie dressings, if you need any at all.
French fries, chips	Baked potato, or mashed potato with PUFA margarine or lowfat spread.
Dill pickle	Fresh lettuce, cucumber or celery.

Refuse:	Choose:
Barbecue sauce or ketchup	Fresh tomato slices.
Cole slaw	Fresh lettuce, barbecued beans or corn on the cob with PUFA margarine.
Tartar sauce, salt	Vinegar or lemon juice.
Ice cream	Ice milk.
Milk shake	Skim milk.
Sweetened soft drinks	Fresh fruit juice, mineral water with twist of lemon.

START COMPLAINING

We don't like to complain, even when we are disturbed about something important. We don't like to "make a fuss," do we? But think of all the fatty foods you still see in supermarkets, fast-food chains, company cafeterias, schools and hospitals.

Speak up and put your views across. Start complaining about all the fat that is in the American diet, insidiously ruining health. Get some action!

In *supermarkets*, if they don't stock a good range of nonfat, lowfat or reduced-fat food items, talk with the manager or write to the store's headquarters if it is part of a larger food chain. To have improvements in food labeling, write to food manufacturers, the Food and Drug Administration, or your local Congressman.

At *work*, talk with the manager of the cafeteria or your union to check on the fat content in meals and snacks; ask for lowfat alternatives.

Too many *schools* around the country continue to serve lunches loaded with saturates. Ask your Parent Teachers' Association or the school-meals organizer why so many fried dishes are served in the school cafeteria, and why greasy potato chips and candy bars are allowed to be sold in vending machines. Talk with the home-economics teachers to make sure that students are taught healthy food shopping and lowfat preparation of foods.

At your local *hospital*, are patients being given lowfat healthy food to speed recovery? Find out from the hospital board or your local public health authority.

In *retirement homes* and *nursing homes*, where you may have an elderly relative or close friend, are meals carefully planned by a dietitian or under good management to provide reduced-fat diets?

7

An A-to-Z Guide To Cutting Fat and Cholesterol

Alcohol. If you must drink, do it in moderation. Alcoholic drinks tend to be high in calories and low in other nutrients.

Avocados. Tasty for salads but higher in fat content than most other salad ingredients. Use sparingly. Fat content can influence flavor. Californian avocados contain 82 percent fat; Florida fruit, 66 percent.

Beans, peas, etc. *See* Legumes.

Breads. Avoid fat-layered croissants, Danish-type breads, cheese-breads, fancy loaves with nuts, and commercial croutons. Check labels for fiber content as some breads are dark merely from caramel coloring. Good choices: wholegrain loaves, plain bagels, plain English muffins, pita bread, flour tortillas and Indian chapatis. Make your own bread stuffing for poultry. Bake your own croutons: spread stale bread cubes on a cookie sheet in a moderate oven and bake for 20 minutes.

Breakfast cereals. Avoid instant oatmeal, commercial mueslis and granolas containing coconut, nuts and added fat. Choose wholegrain, unsugared cereals and top with skim milk and fresh fruit in season. Oatbran cereal can reduce serum cholesterol levels. Wheatbran cereals can remedy constipation and help weight control. Check labels carefully as many cereals, including the trendy oat products, are high in calories and saturated fats such as coconut oil.

Butter. Use sparingly. Whip to increase volume, adding a little skim milk or warm water to make it "creamier." Or mix butter with an equal amount of buttermilk for a reduced-calorie spread. For a substitute spread, whirl lowfat cottage cheese in a blender until smooth. Or switch to PUFA margarine and diet spreads. Spread thinly on thick slices of wholegrain breads.

Buttermilk. Despite its fatty-sounding name, buttermilk contains little or no butterfat.

Cakes. Avoid puff-pastry slices, doughnuts, and cream-filled types. If using a commercial cake mix, choose one that allows you to add the fat, so you can use a healthful oil and control the amount. Use nonstick pans to avoid greasing with unnecessary fat. Good choices: light angel-food sponges, Swiss rolls filled with jam (no cream) and meringues. Avoid fatty frostings; make light glazes with confectioners powdered sugar thinned with skim milk.

Candies and confectionery. Eat in moderation to avoid "empty calories." Avoid chocolate with its highly-saturated cocoa butter, and cream toffees. Minimum-fat candies: plain peppermints, marshmallows, hard candies, gumdrops and jelly beans.

Cheeses. Generally high in saturated fat. Look for labels with "reduced fat," "half fat" or "contains 40 percent less fat," and varieties made with lowfat milk. Fresh cheese usually has less fat and fewer calories than aged cheese. Slice cheese thinly instead of having a big chunk. Use less cheese than recipes specify. Use no salt in recipes containing cheese. Check labels on cream cheese — some can substitute for butter as a spread, halving fat and calories. Make a low-calorie cream cheese with nonfat plain yogurt, straining for about five hours or overnight through a coffee-maker cone lined with filter-paper.

Chocolate. Usually saturated fat in the cocoa butter, plus palm oil or coconut oil. Bars of nut chocolate can be 60 percent fat. Avoid imitation chocolate chips made with highly-saturated palm kernel oil. Plain cocoa powder has little fat; carob powder is lowfat. Substitute these in baking, candy-making and chocolate drinks. *See* also Candies and confectionery.

Coffee creamers and whiteners. Read package labels. Dairy creamers are obviously highly-saturated. Imitation (nondairy) products are often higher in fat than their natural counterparts, with highly-saturated coconut or palm oils. Substitute skim or lowfat milk, evaporated skim milk or nonfat powdered milk.

Condiments. Avoid mayonnaise, tartar sauce and creamed horseradish. Create your own horseradish "cream" with nonfat plain yogurt.

Cookies. Check commercial labels. High-fat varieties are shortbreads, butter cookies, and those containing peanut butter and nuts or savory biscuits containing cheese. Lower-fat varieties: fig bars, gingersnaps and sponge fingers.

Crackers. Check labels. Puff varieties may have high fat content. Lowfat varieties may include unsalted saltines, crispbreads, breadsticks, matzos, Melba toast and rice cakes.

Cream. Highly-saturated fat. Food companies may also add emulsifiers and stabilizers such as mono- and diglycerides, to give a longer shelf-life. Use sparingly; keep for special occasions only. For a nonfat dessert topping, beat nonfat dried milk with ice water until it reaches the soft-peak stage, then add a spoonful of lemon juice and beat until stiff. Or use evaporated skim milk. Cook old-fashioned custard sauce using skim milk, cornstarch, a small dash of sugar and a choice of flavoring – no egg.

Desserts. Evaluate your old recipes to reduce fats and sugar without compromising style. Abandon rich cheesecakes and tortes in favor of fresh whole fruit, fruit salads, gelatins, sherbets, ice milk, lowfat yogurt, frozen yogurt and puddings made with skim milk.

Dips. Avoid ready-made dips using sour cream and mayonnaise. Substitute nonfat plain yogurt seasoned with Dijon mustard.

Eggplant (aubergine). To reduce the amount of oil absorbed during cooking, sprinkle thin slices of raw eggplant with salt, drain in a colander for 30 minutes. Rinse well, pat dry, brush with a smear of oil, then bake.

Eggs. An egg a day for breakfast could spell disaster for the heart-conscious. Eat no more than two or three eggs per week, including those used in baked products and other dishes containing eggs. Buy smaller-sized or reduced-cholesterol eggs. As cholesterol is concentrated in the yolks, use egg whites only, doubling the quantity required in recipes. If a recipe specifies one whole egg, use two egg whites instead. Egg substitutes are mostly egg whites. Check brand labels for fat, calorie and sodium content.

Fats. Use all fats and oils sparingly. Avoid animal-origin fats including lard, chicken fat, beef suet and tallow, mutton fat, bacon- and meat-drippings. Also highly-saturated cocoa butter (used in chocolate) and tropical oils (coconut, palm and palm-kernel) often used in baked products, nondairy creamers, whipped toppings, ice-cream toppings, candies and commercially-fried foods. Heart-healthy alternatives: PUFA vegetable oils, soft margarines and diet spreads.

Fiber. Fiber is found in fruits, vegetables, whole grains and legumes − none in meat or milk products. Fiber can be water-soluble or water-insoluble; it's good to have some of both. Most people can benefit by having between 25 and 35 grams of dietary fiber each day; not more than 35g daily because of possible harmful effects. Water-soluble fiber has gums and pectins which dissolve to form gel-like substances effective in reducing the body's absorption of fat, lowering cholesterol and triglycerides, and losing weight. It can reduce sugar absorption and improve mineral absorption. Examples: oatbran, oatmeal, dried beans, dried peas, apples and citrus fruits. On the other hand, water-insoluble fiber cannot be dissolved in water nor broken down by digestive enzymes, but it can absorb water, swell up and add bulk. It protects against digestive tract problems. It keeps food moving along, so helps reduce the risk of colon cancers, remedies constipation and helps with weight loss, but may cause mineral loss. Examples: whole grains, wheatbran and whole-wheat breakfast cereals.

Fish. Eat fish at least twice a week. Select fresh or frozen cod, haddock, halibut, perch and sole. Bake fillets in aluminum foil with a little wine and herbs. Avoid ready-prepared fish with batter coatings, breadcrumbs, butter and cream sauces. Avoid tuna and sardines packed in oil. Water-packed tuna has two-thirds less fat than oil-packed. If water-packed tuna is un-obtainable, rinse oil-packed tuna to remove excess oil before eating. If water-packed sardines are hard to find, those packed in tomato- or mustard-sauce have fewer fat calories but sodium levels may be high. Canned salmon can range in color from red to pale pink. The deeper the red, the higher the fat content. Avoid fish roe including caviar!

Fruits. Healthy fast foods since the Garden of Eden. Try to have five servings of fruit (or vegetables) each day. Few fruits have fat unless it is added during cooking or processing. Coconut is an exception: whether fresh or shredded, coconut and coconut products are high in fat and the fat is packed with saturates. Deep orange and yellow fruits, such as apricots and peaches, are rich in beta-carotene, which may reduce your risk of certain cancers. Pectins found in many fruits are a form of fiber that may effectively reduce cholesterol and triglycerides in the blood.

Game. Wild game such as rabbit, pheasant, venison and wild duck generally have less fat than their domesticated counterparts specially raised for the market. Reduced-fat content makes birds less caloric but perhaps less tender. Remove skin from game before cooking to reduce fat content still further. Slow, moist cooking methods such as stewing, covered roasting and braising in broth, juices or wine, are best for leaner, less tender game.

Garlic. Can play an important role in combating high blood pressure and cancer. Fresh garlic makes dishes tasty and healthy. Use garlic powder for quick convenience, but never garlic salt.

Grains. Rice, barley and so on are lowfat food items if cooked without added fat. Choose brown rice for extra fiber. Introduce your family to less common grains such as bulgar. Use as side dishes, pilafs and casserole bases, or toss into hamburgers and meat loaves to "stretch" the meat.

Hydrogenation. Margarines and shortening in commercial baked goods are often heavily hydrogenated. Some critics of hydrogenation claim that the process creates an unnatural form of fat (*trans* fatty acids) with a slightly rearranged chemical structure. *Trans* fats are suspected in the promotion of tumors and have been blamed for contributing to atheromatous plaques, but no complete evidence is available.

Ice cream and **ice milk.** Compare labels of ice creams and frozen custards (soft serve) as premium brands can be fat-loaded and caloric with sweeteners. Look for frozen yogurt, fruit sherbets, or ice milk with fewer fat calories than ice cream.

Legumes. Beans, garbanzos (chickpeas), peas and lentils are economical sources of lowfat protein, serving as good alternatives to high-fat meat. Try adding black beans to rice and soups, garbanzos in salads, kidney beans in chili and salads, lentils in soups, limas in succotash and soups, navy and pink beans in baked-bean dishes, and pinto beans in many Mexican dishes. Salads made with marinated beans can take the place of mayonnaise-laden potato- and macaroni salads and coleslaw; dress lightly with herbed or wine vinegars. *See* also Soy products.

Margarines. Use sparingly. Under Federal law, regular margarine must contain 80 percent fat, spreads 50 to 60 percent fat, and diet margarine 40 percent fat. Always use soft margarine, usually sold in tub containers, or liquid margarine with a high proportion of liquid vegetable oil. Diet margarines contain a high proportion of water, to reduce calories, making them unsuitable for cooking.

Marinades. Marinades can give flavor to cheap, lean, tough meats, but generally they only tenderize the meat they touch, not deeper parts. You don't need oil in marinades. Substitute compatible liquids such as vegetable broth, fat-free stock or cooking wine. Or try nonfat plain yogurt, as featured in many savory East Indian dishes. If your marinade does contain oil, be sure to drain well before cooking and serving.

Mayonnaise. Use in moderation. Because regular mayonnaise by law must have at least 65 percent oil, plus whole eggs and egg yolks, it can be a cholesterol-raising product. Commercial mayonnaise may be thinned with vinegar, lemon juice or tomato juice. Look for reduced-calorie or reduced-fat mayonnaise. Try this cholesterol-watcher's recipe in your blender: process at high speed 2 egg whites, 1 tablespoon lemon juice and a teaspoon Dijon mustard. Slowly drip in 1/2 to 2/3 cup (120ml to 150ml) safflower oil and blend thoroughly; chill until firm.

Meats and meat products. If you eat red meat, have smaller portions than you have now. When shopping, choose meat with the smallest amount of fat marbling, and look for well-trimmed cuts. A carefully trimmed, grilled chop or steak may have only half the number of fat calories compared to one that is left untrimmed and fried. Combine small amounts of meat with large amounts of vegetables, as in Oriental dishes. Processed meat products, such as bologna, frankfurters, liver sausage and luncheon meats are high in saturated fat and cholesterol − best to leave them on the supermarket shelf. Buy reduced-fat luncheon meats and hams, and products processed from turkey meat; or make your own savory spread by mincing leftover meat, chicken or turkey, and moistening with lowfat mayonnaise or yogurt. Hot dogs made from chicken may have less fat than those made with beef or pork; check labels. *See* also Organ meats.

Milk. Whole milk is a high-fat food item. Select nonfat or lowfat milk for table use and in cooking. Evaporated skim milk and buttermilk work well in baking. Make your own evaporated skim milk using nonfat dried milk and half the quantity of water needed to make skim milk. A drop of vanilla essence can make nonfat milk taste rich.

Nuts. Avoid nut snacks that have been roasted with fat and coated heavily with salt and/or caramel. Although they tend to be fatty, nuts are nutritious if eaten in moderate amounts and unsalted. Buy nuts in the shell, to keep you busy shelling them and slow down your intake. Check the less fatty lower-caloried nuts such as chestnuts and water chestnuts (not strictly a nut). *See* also Peanut butter.

Oils. Use all oils sparingly, and remember to store them in the refrigerator. Calorie-wise, it matters little whether you use vegetable oil, regular margarine, butter, lard or suet, but PUFA vegetable oil, olive oil and soft margarine are less damaging to blood vessels. Large amounts of PUFA oils may promote cancer. Liquid oils are processed to make their smoke point as high as possible, making them better choices for cooking. Safflower, soybean, cottonseed and corn oils have higher smoking points than peanut and sesame oils. Avoid highly-saturated coconut, palm and palm-kernel oils, commonly used in commercial baked products and candies.

Organ meats. To reduce cholesterol intake, have heart, liver, kidney and sweetbreads only occasionally. Tongue has no more cholesterol than other meats, but is high in saturated fat, so reserve it for special occasions.

Pastas. Use instead of meat in casseroles to reduce fat and cholesterol. Choose wholegrain pastas for significantly larger amounts of fiber. Egg noodles may contain cholesterol. Add pastas to soups, and mix with bread or rice stuffing for poultry. Toss cooked pastas into vinegar and then into salads for a hearty addition.

Peanut butter. Use in moderation. Most peanut butters are salted, sugared and laced with hydrogenated (saturated) vegetable oil. Look for "natural" peanut butter made from 100 percent peanuts. If not in your supermarket, try health-food shops. Or buy peanuts and grind your own in blender or food processor.

Pies. Avoid flaky or puff pastry. Commercial pies and prebaked piecrusts usually have cholesterol-raising fats. Make crumb crusts instead of traditional pastry dough. Or make short-crust pastry with PUFA oil. Instead of two-crust pies, make flans and open tarts. Instead of pies with fat-rich crusts, substitute fruit cobblers baked with toppings of raw oatmeal or oat cereal.

Potatoes. Boiled potatoes contain no fat; French fries are 45 percent fat; chips, 60 percent. Baked potatoes are not fattening unless you put high-fat extras on them. Top jacket potatoes with nonfat yogurt, flavored vinegars, curry powder, fresh black pepper, lemon juice, stewed tomatoes or Mexican salsa.

Poultry. White meats such as chicken and turkey contain more PUFA than any other meats. Light meat has less fat than dark portions. Discard skin of poultry before cooking and you remove 50 percent of the fat. Avoid duck and goose which are more fatty, even when skinned. Avoid deep-frying. "Fry" chicken in the oven with your own coating of fine breadcrumbs and herbs. Never buy a prebasted roasting bird – it will have been pumped full of fat, sodium and unnatural chemicals. Make your own poultry dressing, baking it in a separate dish, using fat-free broth to moisten. If stuffing is put inside birds, too much fat is absorbed. Baste birds with broth, fruit juice or wine instead of butter, bacon fat or oil.

Preserves. Jams, jellies and marmalade are low in fat, but use in moderation. Avoid egg-based lemon curd spread.

Salad dressings. Use in moderation. Many dressings are high in saturates and sodium. Thin commercial dressings with vinegar, lemon juice or tomato juice. Try commercial reduced-calorie or no-oil dressings. Make your own dressings, using some of the flavorful vinegars, plus herbs, spices, vegetable broth or defatted chicken broth.

Salads. Can be a great way to increase fiber and vitamins into your diet, but use avocados sparingly and keep dressings to a minimum. Avoid prepacked coleslaw and potato salad. Make your own, tossed lightly with nonfat plain yogurt.

Salt and **salt-substitutes**. Shake the salt habit! No more salt at table or in cooking. Spark flavors with fresh or dried herbs, lemon juice, fresh garlic or finely-chopped onion. Avoid monosodium glutamate, baking powder and garlic salt. Cut down on Worcestershire sauce, steak sauce, soy sauce and tomato ketchup. Salt-substitutes are not for everyone. Check with your doctor if you have kidney problems, as substitutes frequently contain potassium.

Sandwiches. Resolve to make leaner sandwiches for brown-bag lunches. Diet spreads instead of butter or margarine; wholegrain breads instead of white; a dressing of French mustard or nonfat yogurt instead of mayonnaise. Cut back on luncheon sausage and high-fat cheeses. Choose sliced turkey, chicken or tuna, or sandwiches of bean sprouts, tomatoes, cucumbers and lettuce. If you must have luncheon meat, make it one slice instead of two; a half-sandwich instead of a whole one. Routinely put fresh fruits into packed lunches.

Sauces. Those made with fats can double or triple the calorie count of a dish. Consider simply drizzling lemon juice over steamed vegetables instead of a high-fat cheese sauce. If making Béchamel or white sauce, use nonfat milk rather than cream or whole milk. Season well with herbs, curry powder, lemon juice or a little white wine.

Sausages. Usually with a high-fat content and to be avoided or only eaten occasionally. If you must buy them, prick well before grilling, to release the maximum amount of fat. Look for reduced-fat products.

Smoked foods. Most hams and bacon are high-fat and high-sodium. Check labels and look for reduced-fat products. Eat in moderation to reduce exposure to nitrates, sodium compounds and other chemicals.

Snacks. Some snacks cooked in oil may be 40 percent fat. Avoid potato chips, corn chips and roasted nuts. Movie theaters often use coconut oil when preparing popcorn; take your own plain unbuttered popcorn to the show. Instead of buying tortilla chips, cut fresh ones and bake instead of fry. Nibble on plain unsalted crackers, vegetable sticks, cherry-sized tomatoes and fresh fruit. Replace junk snacks with nutritious ones that are handy to eat.

Soups. Avoid cream soups, vichysoisse and chunky style with large amounts of meat. If you must buy commercial cream soups, reconstitute with nonfat milk or milk/water. Make clear soups and broths, thickened if necessary with a purée of vegetables or breadcrumbs. Substitute all or part of meat in soups with dried beans or lentils for heart-saving heartiness. Prepare soup overnight and skim off all congealed fat on top before reheating.

Sour cream. Substitute plain nonfat yogurt whenever possible, for dips and toppings. For topping baked potatoes, blend reduced-fat cottage cheese with a spoonful of nonfat yogurt, and season with fresh garlic, chives or herbs, or try Mexican salsa.

Soy products. You may be more familiar with products derived from soy beans rather than the beans themselves: soy sauce, soy flour, tofu and textured vegetable protein. Tofu is cheese-like curds that can replace fatty meat or cheese. Tofu is high-calcium, high-protein, cholesterol-free and low in sodium. Crumble it into soups and salads; dice finely and stir-fry with vegetables.

Sugar. Use in moderation. Much of the sugar we eat is no longer brought home in a bag. Food manufacturers add sugar to many products you wouldn't think were sweet: ketchup, tomato sauce, pickles, soups and spaghetti sauces. Select brands that do not have added sugar.

Vegetables. Avoid frozen vegetables in cream sauces or butter sauces. Put crunchy raw vegetables into salads. They take longer to eat, and chewing makes them satisfying. Dress leftover vegetables with vinegar and toss into salads. Sauté vegetables in a small amount of broth instead of oil. Thicken soups with puréed vegetables instead of cream. Stuff fish and poultry with vegetables instead of breadcrumbs.

Vegetarianism. Try vegetarian meals at least once a week, every week. Don't substitute meat with high-fat cheeses or high-cholesterol eggs.

Vinegars. Collect distinctive gourmet vinegars (balsamic, herbal, fruit-flavored) and use them without oil in dressings and marinades.

Whipped butter, whipped margarine. Air is beaten in for easy spreading. They may have one-third fewer calories than regular butter or margarine.

Yogurt. Use nonfat plain yogurt instead of sour cream for topping baked potatoes. For sweet yogurt, buy plain yogurt and add chopped fruits or a teaspoon of preserves. Frozen yogurt may be low in fat, but beware added calories from rich chocolate or carob coatings and added sugar. For a tangy salad dressing, mix yogurt with fruit juice or vinegar. Toss yogurt instead of mayonnaise into potato salad, pasta salad, Russian salad and vegetable salad.

Zabaglione. A high-cholesterol dessert to be avoided.

Zest. Lemon rind to give zip and flavoring to vegetables, fruits and dressings, in place of salt.

Appendix I

Principal Fats and Oils and Their Sources

Fat or oil	Source	Remarks	Cholesterol?
Almond oil	Produced from the nuts of sweet almonds, *Prunus dulcis*, grown in Mediterranean-type climates.	Mostly mono-unsaturated.	No
Arachis oil	*See* Peanut oil.		
Avocado oil	Oil produced from avocados, *Persea americana*, also known as alligator pears.	Mostly mono-unsaturated.	No
Benne oil	*See* Sesame oil.		
Borneo tallow	"Green butter" produced from kernels of an East Indian and Malaysian plant, *Shorea stenoptera*.	Closely akin to cocoa butter, and eaten in countries that produce it.	No
Butter	Produced by churning cows' milk or cream.	Largely saturated fat. Contains substantial amounts of vitamins A and D, calcium and phosphorus.	Yes

Fat or oil	Source	Remarks	Cholesterol?
Canola oil (also known as rapeseed or colza oil)	Produced from the pressed seeds of rape plants, *Brassica napus*, a member of the mustard family.	Mostly monounsaturated. High in omega-3 PUFAs for averting abnormal blood clotting.	No
Castor oil (also known as ricinus oil)	Extracted from seeds of the castor bean, *Ricinus communis*, one of the spurge family.	Formerly used as a cathartic, but now considered harmful for internal use. Used primarily in industry.	No
Cocoa butter (also known as theobroma oil)	Obtained from cacao or cocoa beans, *Theobroma cacao*.	Mostly saturated. One of the most stable fats known, cocoa butter contains antioxidants discouraging rancidity, allowing storage life of 2 to 5 years. Used with other fats to improve their stability. Important component in chocolate.	No
Coconut oil	Vegetable oil extracted from copra or dried kernel meat of coconut palms, *Cocos nucifera*. One of the world's largest sources of edible oil.	92 percent saturated. Widely used in food manufacturing and commercial frying.	No
Cod liver oil	Obtained from the livers of cod, *Gadus morrhua*, and related fish.	A typical marine-animal oil. Good source of vitamins A and D. High in PUFAs. Easily subject to rancidity. Often sold as a health supplement.	Yes
Colza oil	*See* Canola oil.		

Fat or oil	Source	Remarks	Cholesterol?
Corn oil	Obtained from the seed kernels of Indian corn or maize, *Zea mays*.	Mostly polyunsaturated. Large quantities converted to margarine by hydrogenation.	No
Cottonseed oil	Extracted from the seed kernels of the cotton plant, *Gossypium hirsutum*.	Polyunsaturated. Widely used for salad dressings and in cooking. For shortening and margarine, oil is partially hardened by hydrogenation, thus chemically converting part of the unsaturated fatty acids to saturated.	No
Diet spreads	Various.	Varying blends of oils and fats depending upon availability of ingredients. Often contain water and buttermilk to reduce calories, and whipped to introduce air to increase volume.	Maybe
Dripping	Fat drained from meat during cooking.	Saturated. Often used as cooking fat.	Yes
Evening primrose oil	Extracted from the seeds of the evening primrose, *Oenothera biennis*, growing naturally in North America and Britain, and now cultivated in U.S.A., Canada and Europe.	High in polyunsaturates. Widely sold as a health supplement, as a source of gamma linolenic acid.	No

Fat or oil	Source	Remarks	Cholesterol?
Fish oil	Extracted from the livers of fish such as dogfish, halibut, mackerel, rockfish, seabass, soupfin sharks, swordfish, tuna; and from the bodies of anchovies, herring, menhaden and sardines.	Mostly unsaturated. High in omega-3 fatty acids, for averting abnormal blood clotting. Often sold in capsule form as a health supplement.	Yes
Flaxseed oil	*See* Linseed oil.		
Garlic oil	Produced from the bulbs of the garlic plant, *Allium sativum.*	High concentration, usually in capsule form, sold as a health supplement.	No
Ghee (also ghi)	Clarified butter. The name for butterfat used in large quantities on the Indian sub-continent where it is commonly mixed with milkfat of the buffalo.	Mostly saturated fats. Does not become rancid as readily as butter and can be stored unrefrigerated for several months.	Yes
Green butter	*See* Borneo tallow.		
Groundnut oil	*See* Peanut oil.		
Illupi or illipe butter (also mowrah butter)	Hard fat produced from nuts of various East Indian trees of the genus *Madhuca.*	Used occasionally in the chocolate industry. Mostly saturated.	No
Lard	Obtained by rendering fat from pork.	Mostly saturated. Solid or semi-solid. Frequently modified by blending or hydrogenation. Antioxidants usually added to protect against rancidity.	Yes

Fat or oil	Source	Remarks	Cholesterol?
Lecithin (*See* also Soybean oil)	Obtained from the seeds of the soy plant.	High in omega-3 PUFAs. Usually sold as a health supplement.	No
Lemon oil	Obtained from the rinds of lemons, *Citrus limonia*, with flavor sometimes enhanced by adding citral oil from lemon grass, *Cymbopogon citratus*.	Used as food flavoring and in medicines.	No
Linseed oil (also known as flaxseed oil)	Pressed from the seeds of a variety of flax, *Linum usitatissimum*, cultivated mainly in U.S.A., Argentina, Canada and U.S.S.R.	Linseed was used by Ancient Greeks and Romans as a food. Now used as livestock feed. Oil used in industry and not for dietary use.	No
Liquid paraffin	*See* Mineral oil.		
Lowfat spreads	*See* Diet spreads.		
Margarines	Various.	Varying blends of oils and fats depending on availability of ingredients, thus a variable fatty acid composition. Can be hard or soft, with varying degrees of hydrogenation.	Maybe
Mineral oil (also known as liquid paraffin or liquid petrolatum)	Obtained from petroleum by distillation.	Highly refined oil used in medicine as a laxative, but not for culinary use.	No
Mowrah butter	*See* Illupi.		

Fat or oil	Source	Remarks	Cholesterol?
Olive oil	Pressed from mature olives, *Olea europaea*, grown mainly in Mediter-ranean-type climates such as Spain and Italy.	Mostly monounsaturates. Three main grades: extra virgin, fine virgin and virgin (sometimes "pure.")	No
Palm oil	Produced from the pulp of the fruit and seed kernels of the African oil palm, *Elaeis guineensis*, or from the seeds of the cohune palm, *Attalea cohune*.	High in saturates. Widely used in food manufacturing and for commercial frying.	No
Peanut oil (also known as groundnut oil or arachis oil)	Obtained by crushing and extraction from peanuts (also known as groundnuts or earthnuts), *Arachis hypogaea*. Not a true nut, but the pod of an under-ground legume.	Mostly mono-unsaturated.	No
Rapeseed oil	*See* Canola oil.		
Ricinus oil	*See* Castor oil.		
Safflower oil	Obtained from the seeds of the annual thistle-like safflower plant, *Carthamus tinctorius*, grown mostly in U.S.A., Canada, India, Israel, Turkey and Australia.	Highly regarded for its extremely high prop-ortion of PUFAs.	No
Salad oil (and cooking oil)	Various, including corn, cottonseed, olive, peanut, safflower, soybean and sunflower oils.	Blend of different oils, depending on availability of ingred-ients and flavor desired by food manufacturers. May undergo light hydrogenation.	No

Fat or oil	Source	Remarks	Cholesterol?
Schmaltz	Fat or grease rendered from chicken and other poultry.	Mostly saturated fats. Used in Jewish cooking.	Yes
Sesame oil (also known as benne oil)	Expressed from seeds of the annual sesame plant, *Sesamum indicum*.	Mostly PUFAs. This oil resists rancidity. Used in salad and cooking oils, in shortenings and margarines.	No
Shea butter	Hard fat produced from shea nuts, the seeds of the shea tree, *Butyrospermum parkii*, grown in West Africa.	Occasionally used as a component of confectionery fats.	No
Shortening	Various.	Can be made from several fats and oils, depending on availability of ingredients. Usually some hydrogenation.	Maybe
Soybean oil (also known as soyabean or sojabean)	Obtained from the seeds of the soy plant, *Glycine max.* or *Glycine soja*, an annual legume.	Mostly polyunsaturated fats. The oil is frequently processed into margarine, shortening and vegetarian cheeses.	No
Suet	Hard fat produced from beef, mutton, etc. and processed to yield tallow.	Highly saturated.	Yes
Sunflower oil	Compressed from the seeds of certain species of sunflower plants, *Helianthus annuus*, cultivated in U.S.A., U.K., Egypt, India and U.S.S.R.	Mostly polyunsaturated fats.	No

Fat or oil	Source	Remarks	Cholesterol?
Tallow (animal source)	Extracted by cutting and boiling the hard fat from beef, mutton and horse-meat.	Mostly saturated.	Yes
Theobroma oil	*See* Cocoa butter.		
Vegetable oil	Various. May include coconut, corn, cotton-seed, palm, safflower, soybean and sunflower oils.	Can be a blend of different oils depending on availability of ingredients. If it contains coconut or palm oil, it will have a high proportion of saturates. May undergo hydrogenation to produce solid shortening with even higher saturation.	No
Walnut oil (also butternut)	Expressed from the sweet oily nuts of black walnut trees, *Juglans nigra*, or butternut trees, *Jicinerea*	Mostly PUFAs.	No
Wheat germ oil	Produced from the kernels of whole wheat grain of the genus *Triticum*.	Mostly PUFA. Can quickly become rancid.	No

Appendix II

Burning Up The Fat:
Calories Used
During Exercise

Calories * used per hour	Activity	Benefits
72 - 84	Lying down, sleeping, sitting, talking.	No conditioning value.
120 - 150	Walking, 1 to 2 mph.	Insufficiently strenuous unless your capacity for exercise is very limited.
150 - 240	Golf, using a powered cart.	Insufficiently strenuous or continuous to promote endurance.
240 - 300	Housework (cleaning windows, mopping floors, vacuuming).	Adequate for conditioning if carried out continuously for 20 to 30 minutes.

* Note: These figures are based on a person weighing 150 pounds (68kg). The figures will be higher for those who weigh more; lower for those who weigh less.

173

Calories used per hour	Activity	Benefits
240 - 300	Bowling.	Too intermittent. Insufficient to promote endurance.
	Walking, 3 mph, bicycling, 6 mph.	Adequate conditioning if your capacity is limited.
	Golf, pulling cart.	Useful for conditioning if you walk briskly.
300 *	Swimming.	Beneficial.
300 - 360	Housework (scrubbing floors), calisthenics, ballet exercises.	Adequate endurance if carried out in at least 2-minute periods.
	Walking, 3.5 mph, bicycling, 8 mph.	Usually good dynamic aerobic exercise.
	Table tennis, badminton, volleyball.	Vigorous continuous play can have endurance benefits.
	Tennis, doubles.	Not very beneficial unless play is continuous for at least 2 minutes at a time.
350 - 420	Walking, 4 mph, bicycling, 10 mph.	Beneficial.
	Ice- or roller-skating	Skating should be continuous.

* Wide caloric range depending on skill of swimmer, stroke, pace maintained, water temperature, body composition, water currents, and other factors.

Calories used per hour	Activity	Benefits
400	Heavy gardening work, ditch digging with hand shovel.	Endurance-building if continuous, rhythmic and repetitive.
420 - 480	Walking, 5 mph, bicycling, 11 mph.	Beneficial.
	Tennis, singles.	Beneficial, if played 30 minutes or more with an attempt to keep moving.
	Water skiing.	Very risky for people with high risk of heart disease or others out of condition.
480 - 600	Jogging, 5 mph, bicycling, 12 mph.	Beneficial, endurance-building.
	Downhill skiing.	Too short to promote significant endurance. Combination of stress from altitude, cold and exercise may be too great for some people with cardiovascular disease.
600 - 650	Running, 5.5 mph, bicycling, 13 mph.	Excellent conditioner.
Above 660	Running, 6 mph or more.	Excellent conditioner.

Adapted from *Beyond Diet - Exercise Your Way to Fitness and Heart Health* (CPC International) and *Basic Bodywork for Fitness and Health* (American Medical Association).

Appendix III

Food, Fats and Cholesterol

Item	Food	Energy	Total Fat	Fatty Acids Satu-rated	Fatty Acids Mono-unsat.	Fatty Acids Poly-unsat.	Chol-est.
		kcal	*grams*	*grams*	*grams*	*grams*	*mg*
DAIRY PRODUCTS:							
	Butter. *See* item 46 in Fats and Oils.						
	Cheese:						
	American:						
1.	Processed (1 oz)	105	9	5.6	2.5	0.3	27
2.	Cheese food (1 oz)	95	7	4.4	2.0	0.2	18
3.	Cheese spread (1 oz)	80	6	3.8	1.8	0.2	16
4.	Blue (1 oz)	100	8	5.3	2.2	0.2	21
5.	Camembert (1 1/3 oz)	115	9	5.8	2.7	0.3	27
6.	Cheddar (1 oz)	115	9	6.0	2.7	0.3	30
7.	Cottage, lowfat, 2% (1 cup)	205	4	2.8	1.2	0.1	19
8.	Cream (1 oz)	100	10	6.2	2.8	0.4	31
9.	Mozzarella, part skim (1 oz)	80	5	3.1	1.4	0.1	15

Note: Calories have been rounded to the nearest 5 calories. Values for fat are derived from specific factors in the Atwater System (for example, 8.37 calories per gram of fat in fruit, 8.79 calories per gram of fat in milk, and 9.02 calories per gram of fat in meats and animal fats), and rounded to whole numbers. Most nutrition labeling uses an average of 9 calories per gram of fat.

Item	Food	Energy	Total Fat	Fatty Acids Satu- rated	Mono- unsat.	Poly- unsat.	Chol- est.
		kcal	*grams*	*grams*	*grams*	*grams*	*mg*
10.	Parmesan (1 oz)	130	9	5.4	2.5	0.2	22
11.	Ricotta,						
	part skim (1 cup)	340	19	12.1	5.7	0.6	76
12.	Swiss (1 oz)	105	8	5.0	2.1	0.3	26
	Cream, imitation:						
13.	Powdered (1 tsp)	10	1	0.7	tr	tr	0
14.	Sour (1 tbsp)	20	2	1.6	0.2	0.1	1
15.	Cream, sour (1 tbsp)	25	3	1.6	0.7	0.1	5
	Cream, sweet:						
16.	Half & half (1 tbsp)	20	2	1.1	0.5	0.1	6
17. —	Whipped topping,						
	pressurized (1 tbsp)	10	1	0.4	0.2	tr	2
	Whipping:						
18.	Heavy (1 tbsp)	50	6	3.5	1.6	0.2	21
19.	Light (1 tbsp)	45	5	2.9	1.4	0.1	17
	Ice cream, vanilla:						
	Regular, 11% fat						
20.	(1 cup)	270	14	8.9	4.1	0.5	59
21.	Rich, 16% fat (1 cup)	350	24	14.7	6.8	0.9	88
22.	Soft serve (1 cup)	375	23	13.5	6.7	1.0	153
23.	Ice milk, 4% fat						
	(1 cup)	185	6	3.5	1.6	0.2	18
	Milk:						
24.	Buttermilk (1 cup)	100	2	1.3	0.6	0.1	9
25.	Lowfat, 1% (1 cup)	105	2	1.5	0.7	0.1	10
26.	Lowfat, 2% (1 cup)	125	5	2.9	1.4	0.2	18
27.	Nonfat, skim (1 cup)	90	1	0.4	0.2	tr	5
28.	Whole, 3.3% (1 cup)	150	8	5.1	2.4	0.3	33
	Milk, canned:						
29.	Condensed (1 cup)	980	27	16.8	7.4	1.0	104
	Evaporated:						
30.	Skim (1 cup)	200	1	0.3	0.2	tr	9
31.	Whole (1 cup)	340	19	11.6	5.9	0.6	74
32.	Milk, dried, nonfat,						
	made-up (1 cup)	245	tr	0.3	0.1	tr	12
	Milk beverages:						
33.	Choc. milk (1 cup)	210	8	5.3	2.5	0.3	31

Item	Food	Energy	Total Fat	Fatty Acids Satu-rated	Mono-unsat.	Poly-unsat.	Chol-est.
		kcal	*grams*	*grams*	*grams*	*grams*	*mg*
34.	Cocoa, with whole milk (1 cup)	225	9	5.4	2.5	0.3	33
35.	Eggnog, coml. (1 cup)	340	19	11.3	5.7	0.9	149
36.	Milk shake, thick, vanilla (10 oz)	315	9	5.3	2.5	0.3	33
37.	Sherbet (1 cup)	270	4	2.4	1.1	0.1	14
	Yogurt:						
38.	With milk solids, nonfat (1 cup)	125	tr	0.3	0.1	tr	4
39.	Without solids, whole milk (1 cup)	140	7	4.8	2.0	0.2	29
EGGS:							
	Eggs, large, cooked:						
40.	Fried in butter (1 egg)	95	7	2.7	2.7	0.8	278
41.	Poached (1 egg)	80	6	1.7	2.2	0.7	273
42.	Scrambled, with milk & butter (1 egg)	110	8	3.2	2.9	0.8	282
	Eggs, large, raw:						
43.	Whole (1 egg)	80	6	1.7	2.2	0.7	274
44.	White (1 white)	15	tr	0.0	0.0	0.0	0
45.	Yolk (1 yolk)	65	6	1.7	2.2	0.7	272
FATS AND OILS:							
46.	Butter (1 tbsp)	100	11	7.1	3.3	0.4	31
47.	Fat, cooking, vegetable (1 tbsp)	115	13	3.3	5.8	3.4	0
48.	Lard (1 tbsp)	115	13	5.1	5.9	1.5	12
	Margarine:						
49.	Imitation, 40% fat, soft (1 tbsp)	50	5	1.1	2.2	1.9	0
	Regular, 80% fat:						
50.	hard (1 tbsp)	100	11	2.2	5.0	3.6	0
51.	soft (1 tbsp)	100	11	1.9	4.0	4.8	0
	Spread, 60% fat:						
52.	hard (1 tbsp)	75	9	2.0	3.6	2.5	0
53.	soft (1 tbsp)	75	9	1.8	4.4	1.9	0

Item	Food	Energy	Total Fat	Fatty Acids Satu-rated	Fatty Acids Mono-unsat.	Fatty Acids Poly-unsat.	Chol-est.
		kcal	grams	grams	grams	grams	mg
	Oils, salad/cooking:						
54.	Corn (1 tbsp)	125	14	1.8	3.4	8.2	0
55.	Olive (1 tbsp)	125	14	1.9	10.3	1.2	0
56.	Peanut (1 tbsp)	125	14	2.4	6.5	4.5	0
57.	Safflower (1 tbsp)	125	14	1.3	1.7	10.4	0
58.	Soybean-cottonseed blend, hydrogenated (1 tbsp)	125	14	2.5	4.1	6.7	0
59.	Sunflower (1 tbsp)	125	14	1.4	2.7	9.2	0
	Salad dressings:						
60.	Blue cheese (1 tbsp)	75	8	1.5	1.8	4.2	3
	French:						
61.	Low calorie (1 tbsp)	25	2	0.2	0.3	1.0	0
62.	Regular (1 tbsp)	85	9	1.4	4.0	3.5	0
	Italian:						
63.	Low calorie (1 tbsp)	5	tr	tr	tr	tr	0
64.	Regular (1 tbsp)	80	9	1.3	3.7	3.2	0
	Mayonnaise:						
65.	Imitation (1 tbsp)	35	3	0.5	0.7	1.6	4
66.	Regular (1 tbsp)	100	11	1.7	3.2	5.8	8
	Thousand Island:						
67.	Low calorie (1 tbsp)	25	2	0.2	0.4	0.9	2
68.	Regular (1 tbsp)	60	6	1.0	1.3	3.2	4
69.	Vinegar & oil, home recipe (1 tbsp)	70	8	1.5	2.4	3.9	0
	FISH AND SHELLFISH:						
70.	Clams, canned (3 oz)	85	2	0.5	0.5	0.4	54
71.	Crab, canned (1 cup)	135	3	0.5	0.8	1.4	135
72.	Fishsticks, frozen (1 fishstick)	70	3	0.8	1.4	0.8	26
73.	Flounder, baked, no added fat (3 oz)	80	1	0.3	0.2	0.4	59
74.	Haddock, breaded, fried (3 oz)	175	9	2.4	3.9	2.4	75
75.	Halibut, broiled, with butter/lemon (3 oz)	140	6	3.3	1.6	0.7	62
76.	Herring, pickled (3 oz)	190	13	4.3	4.6	3.1	85

Item	Food	Energy	Total Fat	Fatty Acids Satu-rated	Mono-unsat.	Poly-unsat.	Chol-est.
		kcal	*grams*	*grams*	*grams*	*grams*	*mg*
	Oysters:						
77.	Raw (1 cup)	160	4	1.4	0.5	1.4	120
78.	Breaded, fried. (1 oyster)	90	5	1.4	2.1	1.4	35
	Salmon:						
79.	Canned, pink (3 oz)	120	5	0.9	1.5	2.1	34
80.	Smoked (3 oz)	150	8	2.6	3.9	0.7	51
81.	Sardines, canned in oil (3 oz)	175	9	2.1	3.7	2.9	85
82.	Scallops, breaded (6 scallops)	195	10	2.5	4.1	2.5	70
	Shrimp:						
83.	Canned (3 oz)	100	1	0.2	0.2	0.4	128
84.	French fried (7 medium, 3 oz)	200	10	2.5	4.1	2.6	168
85.	Sole, baked, no added fat (3 oz)	80	1	0.3	0.2	0.4	59
86.	Trout, broiled, with butter/lemon (3 oz)	175	9	4.1	2.9	1.6	71
	Tuna, canned:						
87.	Oil pack (3 oz)	165	7	1.4	1.9	3.1	55
88.	Water pack (3 oz)	135	1	0.3	0.2	0.3	48
FRUITS AND FRUIT JUICES:							
89.	Apples, raw (1 apple)	80	tr	0.1	tr	0.1	0
90.	Applesauce, canned, sweetened (1 cup)	195	tr	0.1	tr	0.1	0
	Apricots:						
91.	Raw (3 apricots)	50	tr	tr	0.2	0.1	0
92.	Dried (1 cup)	310	1	tr	0.3	0.1	0
	Avocados:						
93.	California (6 oz)	305	30	4.5	19.4	3.5	0
94.	Florida (11 oz)	340	27	5.3	14.8	4.5	0
95.	Bananas (1 banana)	105	1	0.2	tr	0.1	0
96.	Blueberries, raw (1 cup)	80	1	tr	0.1	0.3	0
97.	Cherries, sweet, raw (10 cherries)	50	1	0.1	0.2	0.2	0

Item	Food	Energy	Total Fat	Fatty Acids			Chol-est.
				Satu-rated	Mono-unsat.	Poly-unsat.	
		kcal	grams	grams	grams	grams	mg
	Coconut. *See* item 199 in Legumes, Nuts and Seeds.						
98.	Cranberry sauce, canned (1 cup)	420	tr	tr	0.1	0.2	0
99.	Dates (10 dates)	230	tr	0.1	0.1	tr	0
100.	Figs, dried (10 figs)	475	2	0.4	0.5	0.1	0
101.	Grapefruit, raw (1/2 grapefruit)	40	tr	tr	tr	tr	0
102.	Grapes, Thompson Seedless (10 grapes)	35	tr	0.1	tr	0.1	0
103.	Lemon juice (1 cup)	60	tr	tr	tr	tr	0
104.	Melons, cantaloup (1/2 melon)	95	1	0.1	0.1	0.3	0
105.	Nectarines (1 nectarine)	65	1	0.1	0.2	0.3	0
	Olives, canned:						
106.	Black (2 large)	15	2	0.3	1.3	0.2	0
107.	Green (4 medium)	15	2	0.2	1.2	0.1	0
108.	Oranges (1 orange)	60	tr	tr	tr	tr	0
109.	Orange juice, frozen, diluted (1 cup)	110	tr	tr	tr	tr	0
110.	Peaches, raw (1 peach)	35	tr	tr	tr	tr	0
111.	Pears, raw (1 pear)	100	1	tr	0.1	0.2	0
112.	Pineapple, canned, juice pack (1 cup)	150	tr	tr	tr	0.1	0
113.	Plums, raw (1 plum)	35	tr	tr	0.3	0.1	0
114.	Prunes, dried, cooked, unsweetened (1 cup)	225	tr	tr	0.3	0.1	0
115.	Raspberries, raw (1 cup)	60	1	tr	0.1	0.4	0
116.	Rhubarb, cooked, sweetened (1 cup)	280	tr	tr	tr	0.1	0
117.	Strawberries, raw (1 cup)	45	1	tr	0.1	0.3	0
118.	Watermelon, without rind (1 lb slice)	155	2	0.3	0.2	1.0	0

Item	Food	Energy	Total Fat	Satu-rated	Mono-unsat.	Poly-unsat.	Chol-est.
		kcal	*grams*	*grams*	*grams*	*grams*	*mg*
GRAIN PRODUCTS:							
119.	Bagel, plain (1 bagel)	200	2	0.3	0.5	0.7	0
120.	Biscuits, from mix						
	(1 biscuit)	95	3	0.8	1.4	0.9	tr
	Breads:						
121.	Boston brown,						
	canned (1 slice)	95	1	0.3	0.1	0.1	3
122.	French (1 slice)	100	1	0.3	0.4	0.5	0
123.	Oatmeal (1 slice)	65	1	0.2	0.4	0.5	0
124.	Pita (1 pita)	165	1	0.1	0.1	0.4	0
125.	Pumpernickel						
	(1 slice)	80	1	0.2	0.3	0.5	0
126.	Rye (1 slice)	65	1	0.2	0.3	0.3	0
127.	White (1 slice)	65	1	0.3	0.4	0.2	0
128.	Wholewheat (1 slice)	70	1	0.4	0.4	0.3	0
	Bread stuffing from mix:						
129.	Dry type (1 cup)	500	31	6.1	13.3	9.6	0
130.	Moist type (1 cup)	420	26	5.3	11.3	8.0	67
	Breakfast cereals:						
131.	All-Bran (1 oz)	70	1	0.1	0.1	0.3	0
132.	Cheerios (1 oz)	110	2	0.3	0.6	0.7	0
133.	Corn Flakes (1 oz)	110	tr	tr	tr	tr	0
134.	Cream of Wheat, regular,						
	cooked (1 cup)	140	tr	0.1	tr	0.2	0
135.	Granola, Nature Valley						
	(1 oz)	125	5	3.3	0.7	0.7	0
136.	100% Natural Cereal						
	(1 oz)	135	6	4.1	1.2	0.5	tr
137.	Oatmeal, regular,						
	cooked (1 cup)	145	2	0.4	0.8	1.0	0
138.	Raisin Bran (1 oz)	90	1	0.1	0.1	0.3	0
139.	Shredded Wheat						
	(1 oz)	100	1	0.1	0.1	0.3	0
	Cakes, from mixes:						
140.	Angel food (1 piece)	125	tr	tr	tr	0.1	0
141.	Coffeecake (1 piece)	230	7	2.0	2.8	1.6	47
142.	Devil's food, w/choc.						
	frosting (1 piece)	235	8	3.5	3.2	1.2	37

Item	Food	Energy	Total Fat	Fatty Acids			Chol-est.
				Satu-rated	Mono-unsat.	Poly-unsat.	
		kcal	*grams*	*grams*	*grams*	*grams*	*mg*
143.	Gingerbread (1 piece)	175	4	1.1	1.8	1.2	1
	Cakes, home recipes:						
144.	Carrot, w/cream cheese frosting (1 piece)	385	21	4.1	8.4	6.7	74
145.	Fruit cake (1 piece)	165	7	1.5	3.6	1.6	20
146.	Pound (1 piece)	120	5	1.2	2.4	1.6	32
	Cakes, commercial:						
147.	White, with white frosting (1 piece)	260	9	2.1	3.8	2.6	3
148.	Cheesecake (1 piece)	280	18	9.9	5.4	1.2	170
	Cookies:						
149.	Brownies, w/nuts, home recipe (1 brownie)	95	6	1.4	2.8	1.2	18
150.	Chocolate chip, coml. (4 cookies)	180	9	2.9	3.1	2.6	5
151.	Fig bars (4 bars)	210	4	1.0	1.5	1.0	27
152.	Peanut butter, home recipe (4 cookies)	245	14	4.0	5.8	2.8	22
153.	Shortbread, coml. (4 small cookies)	155	8	2.9	3.0	1.1	27
154.	Corn chips (1 oz)	155	9	1.4	2.4	3.7	0
155.	Corn meal, cooked (1 cup)	120	tr	tr	0.1	0.2	0
	Crackers:						
156.	Cheese (10 crackers)	50	3	0.9	1.2	0.3	6
157.	Graham (2 crackers)	60	1	0.4	0.6	0.4	0
158.	Melba toast (1 piece)	20	tr	0.1	0.1	0.1	0
159.	Saltines (4 crackers)	50	1	0.5	0.4	0.2	4
160.	Snack-type, standard (1 round cracker)	15	1	0.2	0.4	0.1	0
161.	Croissants (1 roll)	235	12	3.5	6.7	1.4	13
162.	Danish pastry, plain (1 pastry)	220	12	3.6	4.8	2.6	49
	Doughnuts:						
163.	Cake type (1 d'nut)	210	12	2.8	5.0	3.0	20
164.	Yeast, glazed (1 doughnut)	235	13	5.2	5.5	0.9	21

| Item | Food | Energy | Total Fat | Fatty Acids | | | Chol-est. |
				Satu-rated	Mono-unsat.	Poly-unsat.	
		kcal	*grams*	*grams*	*grams*	*grams*	*mg*
	Flours:						
165.	All-purpose, sifted (1 cup)	420	1	0.2	0.1	0.5	0
166.	Wholewheat (1 cup)	400	2	0.3	0.3	1.1	0
167.	French toast, home recipe (1 slice)	155	7	1.6	2.0	1.6	112
168.	Macaroni, cooked (1 cup)	190	1	0.1	0.1	0.3	0
	Muffins, commercial:						
169.	Blueberry (1 muffin)	140	5	1.4	2.0	1.2	45
170.	English (1 muffin)	140	1	0.3	0.2	0.3	0
171.	Noodles, egg, cooked (1 cup)	200	2	0.5	0.6	0.6	50
172.	Pancakes, plain, from mix (1 pancake)	60	2	0.5	0.9	0.5	16
	Pies:						
173.	Apple (1 piece)	405	18	4.6	7.4	4.4	0
174.	Blueberry (1 piece)	380	17	4.3	7.4	4.6	0
175.	Custard (1 piece)	330	17	5.6	6.7	3.2	169
176.	Lemon meringue (1 piece)	355	14	4.3	5.7	2.9	143
177.	Pecan (1 piece)	575	32	4.7	17.0	7.9	95
178.	Pumpkin (1 piece)	320	17	6.4	6.7	3.0	109
	Popcorn, popped:						
179.	Air-popped, (1 cup)	30	tr	tr	0.1	0.2	0
180.	Popped in vegetable oil (1 cup)	55	3	0.5	1.4	1.2	0
181.	Pretzels (10 pretzels)	240	2	0.4	0.8	0.6	0
182.	Rice, white, instant, cooked (1 cup)	180	0	0.1	0.1	0.1	0
	Rolls:						
183.	Dinner (1 roll)	85	2	0.5	0.8	0.6	tr
184.	Hamburger (1 bun)	115	2	0.5	0.8	0.6	tr
185.	Spaghetti, cooked (1 cup)	190	1	0.1	0.1	0.3	0
186.	Toaster pastries (1 pastry)	210	6	1.7	3.6	0.4	0
187.	Tortillas, corn, uncooked (1 tortilla)	65	1	0.1	0.3	0.6	0

Item	Food	Energy	Total Fat	Fatty Acids Satu- rated	Mono- unsat.	Poly- unsat.	Chol- est.
		kcal	grams	grams	grams	grams	mg
LEGUMES, NUTS AND SEEDS:							
188.	Almonds (1 oz)	165	15	1.4	9.6	3.1	0
	Beans, dry:						
	Canned:						
189.	Red kidney (1 cup)	230	1	0.1	0.1	0.6	0
190.	Refried (1 cup)	295	3	0.4	0.6	1.4	0
191.	White, w/franks						
	(1 cup)	365	18	7.4	8.8	0.7	30
192.	White, w/pork and tomato						
	sauce (1 cup)	310	7	2.4	2.7	0.7	10
	Cooked:						
193.	Lima (1 cup)	260	1	0.2	0.1	0.5	0
194.	Pinto (1 cup)	265	1	0.1	0.1	0.5	0
	Beans, fresh, Baby Limas.						
	See item 271 in Vegetables.						
195.	Brazil nuts (1 oz)	185	19	4.6	6.5	6.8	0
196.	Cashew nuts, dry						
	roasted (1 oz)	165	13	2.6	7.7	2.2	0
197.	Chestnuts, European						
	(1 cup)	350	3	0.6	1.1	1.2	0
	Chestnuts, water. *See* item						
	316 in Vegetables.						
198.	Chickpeas (garbanzos),						
	cooked (1 cup)	270	4	0.4	0.9	1.9	0
199.	Coconut, dried, sweeten-						
	ed, shredded (1 cup)	470	33	29.3	1.4	0.4	0
200.	Lentils, dry, cooked						
	(1 cup)	215	1	0.1	0.2	0.5	0
201.	Macadamia nuts, roasted						
	in oil (1 oz)	205	22	3.2	17.1	0.4	0
202.	Peanuts, roasted in oil						
	(1 oz)	165	14	1.9	6.9	4.4	0
203.	Peanut butter (1 tbsp)	95	8	1.4	4.0	2.5	0
	Peas, green. *See* item 293						
	in Vegetables.						
204.	Peas, split, dry, cooked						
	(1 cup)	230	1	0.1	0.1	0.3	0
205.	Pecan nuts (1 oz)	190	19	1.5	12.0	4.7	0
206.	Pistachio nuts (1 oz)	165	14	1.7	9.3	2.1	0

				Fatty Acids		
Item	Food	Energy	Total Fat	Satu- rated	Mono- unsat.	Poly- unsat.	Chol- est.
		kcal	grams	grams	grams	grams	mg
207.	Sesame seeds (1 tbsp)	45	4	0.6	1.7	1.9	0
	Soybean products:						
208.	Tofu (4 oz)	85	5	0.7	1.0	2.9	0
209.	Sunflower seeds (1 oz)	160	14	1.5	2.7	9.3	0
210.	Tahini (1 tbsp)	90	8	1.1	3.0	3.5	0
211.	Walnuts, English						
	(1 oz)	180	18	1.6	4.0	11.1	0

MEATS AND MEAT PRODUCTS:

Beef, cooked:

Item	Food	Energy	Total Fat	Satu- rated	Mono- unsat.	Poly- unsat.	Chol- est.
212.	Bottom round, braised,						
	lean (3 oz)	175	8	2.7	3.4	0.3	75
213.	Chuck blade, braised,						
	lean and fat (3 oz)	325	26	10.8	11.7	0.9	87
	Ground beef, broiled:						
214.	Lean (3 oz)	230	16	6.2	6.9	0.6	74
215.	Regular (3 oz)	245	18	6.9	7.7	0.7	76
216.	Heart, braised						
	(3 oz)	150	5	1.2	0.8	1.6	164
217.	Liver, fried (3 oz)	185	7	2.5	3.6	1.3	410
	Roast, oven cooked:						
218.	Rib, lean and fat						
	(3 oz)	315	26	10.8	11.4	0.9	72
219.	Eye of round, lean						
	and fat (3 oz)	205	12	4.9	5.4	0.5	62
220.	Sirloin steak, broiled,						
	lean and fat (3 oz)	240	15	6.4	6.9	0.6	77
221.	Beef, corned, canned						
	(3 oz)	185	10	4.2	4.9	0.4	80
222.	Beef, dried, chipped						
	(2 1/2 oz)	145	4	1.8	2.0	0.2	46
	Lamb, cooked:						
223.	Chop, loin, broiled,						
	lean and fat (3 oz)	235	16	7.3	6.4	1.0	78
224.	Leg, roasted, lean						
	and fat (3 oz)	205	13	5.6	4.9	0.8	78
225.	Rib, roasted, lean						
	and fat (3 oz)	315	26	12.1	10.6	1.5	77

| | | | | Fatty Acids | | | |
| | | | | Satu- | Mono- | Poly- | Chol- |
Item	Food	Energy	Total Fat	rated	unsat.	unsat.	est.
		kcal	*grams*	*grams*	*grams*	*grams*	*mg*
	Pork, cured, cooked:						
	Bacon:						
226.	Canadian (2 slices)	85	4	1.3	1.9	0.4	27
227.	Regular (3 slices)	110	9	3.3	4.5	1.1	16
228.	Ham, canned (3 oz)	140	7	2.4	3.5	0.8	35
229.	Luncheon meat, canned (2 slices)	140	13	4.5	6.0	1.5	26
	Pork, fresh, cooked:						
230.	Chop, loin, broiled, lean and fat (3 oz)	275	19	7.0	8.8	2.2	84
231.	Rib, roasted, lean and fat (3 oz)	270	20	7.2	9.2	2.3	69
	Sausages:						
232.	Bologna (2 slices)	180	16	6.1	7.6	1.4	31
233.	Braunschweiger (2 slices)	205	18	6.2	8.5	2.1	89
234.	Brown-and-serve (1 link)	50	5	1.7	2.2	0.5	9
235.	Frankfurter, beef/pork (1 frankfurter)	145	13	4.8	6.2	1.2	23
	Frankfurter, chicken. *See* item 246 in Poultry.						
236.	Salami, cooked type (2 slices)	145	11	4.6	5.2	1.2	37
237.	Veal, cutlet, braised (3 oz)	185	9	4.1	4.1	0.6	109
MIXED DISHES:							
238.	Beef pot pie, home recipe: (1 piece)	515	30	7.9	12.9	7.4	42
239.	Chicken à la king, home recipe (1 cup)	470	34	12.9	13.4	6.2	221
240.	Chili con carne w/beans, canned (1 cup)	340	16	5.8	7.2	1.0	28
241.	Macaroni and cheese, home recipe (1 cup)	430	22	9.8	7.4	3.6	44
242.	Quiche Lorraine (1 slice)	600	48	23.2	17.8	4.1	285

Item	Food	Energy	Total Fat	Satu- rated	Mono- unsat.	Poly- unsat.	Chol- est.
				Fatty Acids			
		kcal	grams	grams	grams	grams	mg

POULTRY AND POULTRY PRODUCTS:
Chicken:

Item	Food	Energy	Total Fat	Satu- rated	Mono- unsat.	Poly- unsat.	Chol- est.
243.	Breast, fried in batter, with skin (5 oz)	365	18	4.9	7.6	4.3	119
244.	Breast, roasted, with skin (3 oz)	140	3	0.9	1.1	0.7	73
245.	Canned (5 oz)	235	11	3.1	4.5	2.5	88
246.	Frankfurter (1 frankfurter)	115	9	2.5	3.8	1.8	45
247.	Liver, cooked (1 oz)	30	1	0.4	0.3	0.2	126
248.	Duck, roasted, without skin (1/2 duck)	445	25	9.2	8.2	3.2	197
	Turkey, roasted, without skin:						
249.	Dark meat (3 oz)	160	6	2.1	1.4	1.8	72
250.	Light meat (3 oz)	135	3	0.9	0.5	0.7	59

SOUPS, SAUCES AND GRAVIES:
Soups:
Canned, made w/milk:

Item	Food	Energy	Total Fat	Satu- rated	Mono- unsat.	Poly- unsat.	Chol- est.
251.	Cream of Chicken (1 cup)	190	11	4.6	4.5	1.6	27
252.	Cream of Mushroom (1 cup)	205	14	5.1	3.0	4.6	20
	Canned, made w/water:						
253.	Consommé (1 cup)	15	1	0.3	0.2	tr	tr
254.	Tomato (1 cup)	85	2	0.4	0.4	1.0	0
	Sauces:						
255.	Cheese, from mix, made with milk (1 cup)	305	17	9.3	5.3	1.6	53
256.	White, home recipe (1 cup)	395	30	9.1	11.9	7.2	32
	Gravies:						
257.	Beef, canned (1 cup)	125	5	2.7	2.3	0.2	7
258.	Chicken, from dry mix (1 cup)	85	2	0.5	0.9	0.4	3

Item	Food	Energy	Total Fat	Fatty Acids Satu-rated	Fatty Acids Mono-unsat.	Fatty Acids Poly-unsat.	Chol-est.
		kcal	grams	grams	grams	grams	mg

SUGARS, SWEETS AND DESSERTS:

Candy:

Item	Food	Energy	Total Fat	Satu-rated	Mono-unsat.	Poly-unsat.	Chol-est.
259.	Caramels (1 oz)	115	3	2.2	0.3	0.1	1
	Chocolate:						
260.	Baking (1 oz)	145	15	9.0	4.9	0.5	0
261.	Milk with almonds (1 oz)	150	10	4.8	4.1	0.7	5
262.	Sweet, dark (1 oz)	150	10	5.9	3.3	0.3	0
263.	Hard (1 oz)	110	0	0.0	0.0	0.0	0
264.	Jelly beans (1 oz)	105	tr	tr	tr	0.1	0
265.	Custard, baked (1 cup)	305	15	6.8	5.4	0.7	278
266.	Pudding, canned, chocolate (5 oz)	205	11	9.5	0.5	0.1	1
267.	Sugar, white (1 tbsp)	45	0	0.0	0.0	0.0	0
268.	Syrup, chocolate fudge (2 tbsp)	125	5	3.1	1.7	0.2	0

VEGETABLES AND VEGETABLE PRODUCTS:

Item	Food	Energy	Total Fat	Satu-rated	Mono-unsat.	Poly-unsat.	Chol-est.
269.	Artichokes, globe, cooked (1 artichoke)	55	tr	tr	tr	0.1	0
270.	Asparagus, cooked (1 cup)	45	1	0.1	tr	0.2	0
	Beans, dry, limas. *See* item 193 in Legumes.						
271.	Beans, immature, baby limas, cooked (1 cup)	190	1	0.1	tr	0.3	0
272.	Beans,snap, cooked (1 cup)	45	tr	0.1	tr	0.2	0
273.	Bean sprouts, mung, raw (1 cup)	30	tr	tr	tr	0.1	0
274.	Beets, cooked (1 cup)	55	tr	tr	tr	tr	0
275.	Broccoli, cooked (1 cup)	45	tr	0.1	tr	0.2	0
276.	Brussels sprouts, cooked (1 cup)	60	1	0.2	0.1	0.4	0
	Cabbage:						
277.	Red, raw (1 cup)	20	tr	tr	tr	0.1	0
278.	White, cooked (1 cup)	30	tr	tr	tr	0.2	0
279.	Carrots, cooked (1 cup)	70	tr	0.1	tr	0.1	0

				Fatty Acids		
Item	**Food**	**Energy**	**Total Fat**	**Satu-rated**	**Mono-unsat.**	**Poly-unsat.**	**Chol-est.**
		kcal	*grams*	*grams*	*grams*	*grams*	*mg*
280.	Cauliflower, cooked						
	(1 cup)	30	tr	tr	tr	0.1	0
281.	Celery, raw (1 cup)	20	tr	tr	tr	0.1	0
282.	Collards, cooked						
	(1 cup)	25	tr	0.1	tr	0.2	0
283.	Corn, sweet, cooked						
	(1 ear)	85	1	0.2	0.3	0.5	0
284.	Cucumber (8 slices)	5	tr	tr	tr	tr	0
285.	Eggplant, cooked						
	(1 cup)	25	tr	tr	tr	0.1	0
286.	Kale, cooked (1 cup)	40	1	0.1	tr	0.3	0
287.	Lettuce, iceberg (1 cup)	5	tr	tr	tr	0.1	0
288.	Mushrooms, cooked						
	(1 cup)	40	1	0.1	tr	0.3	0
289.	Onions, raw (1 cup)	55	tr	0.1	0.1	0.2	0
290.	Onion rings, breaded,						
	fried (2 rings)	80	5	1.7	2.2	1.0	0
291.	Parsley (10 sprigs)	5	tr	tr	tr	tr	0
292.	Parsnips, cooked						
	(1 cup)	125	tr	0.1	0.2	0.1	0
293.	Peas, green, cooked						
	(1 cup)	125	tr	0.1	tr	0.2	0
	Peas, split. *See* item 204 in Legumes.						
294.	Peppers, sweet, raw						
	(1 pepper)	20	tr	tr	tr	0.2	0
	Potatoes:						
295.	Baked, with skin						
	(1 potato)	220	tr	0.1	tr	0.1	0
296.	French fried						
	(10 fries)	160	8	2.5	1.6	3.8	0
	Potato products:						
297.	Au gratin, from mix						
	(1 cup)	230	10	6.3	2.9	0.3	12
298.	Hash brown (1 cup)	340	18	7.0	8.0	2.1	0
	Mashed:						
299.	Home recipe w/milk						
	& marg. (1 cup)	225	9	2.2	3.7	2.5	4

Item	Food	Energy	Total Fat	Fatty Acids Satu- rated	Mono- unsat.	Poly- unsat.	Chol- est.
		kcal	*grams*	*grams*	*grams*	*grams*	*mg*
300.	Dehydrated flakes w/milk & butter (1 cup)	235	12	7.2	3.3	0.5	29
301.	Potato chips (10 chips)	105	7	1.8	1.2	3.6	0
302.	Potato salad, with mayonnaise (1 cup)	360	21	3.6	6.2	9.3	170
303.	Scalloped, from mix (1 cup)	230	11	6.5	3.0	0.5	27
304.	Pumpkin, canned (1 cup)	85	1	0.4	0.1	tr	0
305.	Radishes (4 radishes)	5	tr	tr	tr	tr	0
306.	Sauerkraut, canned (1 cup)	45	tr	0.1	tr	0.1	0
307.	Spinach, cooked (1 cup)	40	tr	0.1	tr	0.2	0
308.	Spinach souffle (1 cup)	220	18	7.1	6.8	3.1	184
	Squash, cooked:						
309.	Summer (1 cup)	35	1	0.1	tr	0.2	0
310.	Winter (1 cup)	80	1	0.3	0.1	0.5	0
311.	Sweet potatoes, canned (1 cup)	260	1	0.1	tr	0.2	0
312.	Tomatoes, raw (1 tomato)	25	tr	tr	tr	0.1	0
313.	Tomato juice, canned (1 cup)	40	tr	tr	tr	0.1	0
	Tomato products, canned:						
314.	Paste (1 cup)	220	2	0.3	0.4	0.9	0
315.	Sauce (1 cup)	75	tr	0.1	0.1	0.2	0
316.	Turnips, cooked (1 cup)	30	tr	tr	tr	0.1	0
317.	Vegetable juice cocktail, canned (1 cup)	45	tr	tr	tr	0.1	0
318.	Water chestnuts, canned (1 cup)	70	tr	tr	tr	tr	0

Source: U.S. Department of Agriculture *Nutritive Value of Foods*, Home and Garden Bulletin Number 72, revised 1985.

Appendix IV

Fat and Cholesterol in Fast Foods

Food item	Wt.	Energy	Protein	Carb.	Fat	Chol.
	grams	*kcal*	*grams*	*grams*	*grams*	*mg*
KENTUCKY FRIED CHICKEN:						
Original Recipe:						
Wing	56	181	11.8	5.8	12.3	67
Side breast	95	276	20.0	10.1	17.3	96
Center breast	107	257	25.5	8.0	13.7	93
Drumstick	58	147	13.6	3.4	8.8	81
Thigh	96	278	18.0	8.4	19.2	122
Extra Crispy:						
Wing	57	218	11.5	7.8	15.6	63
Side breast	98	354	17.7	17.3	23.7	66
Center breast	120	353	26.9	14.4	20.9	93
Drumstick	60	173	12.7	5.9	10.9	65
Thigh	112	371	19.6	13.8	26.3	121
Kentucky Nuggets (one)	16	46	2.8	2.2	2.9	12
Kentucky Fries	119	268	4.8	33.3	12.8	2
Mashed Potatoes w/Gravy	86	62	2.1	10.3	1.4	1
Chicken Gravy	78	59	2.0	4.4	3.7	2
Buttermilk Biscuit	75	269	5.1	31.6	13.6	1
Potato Salad	90	141	1.8	12.6	9.3	11
Baked Beans	89	105	5.1	18.4	1.2	1
Corn on the Cob	143	176	5.1	31.9	3.1	1
Cole Slaw	79	103	1.3	11.5	5.7	4

Food item	Wt.	Energy	Protein	Carb.	Fat	Chol.
	grams	kcal	grams	grams	grams	mg
McDONALD'S:						
Chicken McNuggets	109	323	19.1	13.7	21.3	73
Hamburger	100	263	12.4	28.3	11.3	29
Cheeseburger	114	328	15.0	28.5	16.0	41
Quarter Pounder	160	427	24.6	29.3	23.5	81
Quarter Pounder w/Cheese	186	525	29.6	30.5	31.6	107
Big Mac	200	570	24.6	39.2	35.0	83
Filet-O-Fish	143	435	14.7	35.9	25.7	45
McD.L.T.	254	680	30.0	40.0	44.0	101
French Fries, regular	68	220	3.0	26.1	11.5	9
Biscuit w/Sausage and Egg	175	585	19.8	36.4	39.9	285
Biscuit w/Bacon,						
Egg and Cheese	145	483	16.5	33.2	31.6	263
Sausage McMuffin	115	427	17.6	30.0	26.3	59
Sausage McMuffin w/Egg	165	517	22.9	32.2	32.9	287
Egg McMuffin	138	340	18.5	31.0	15.8	259
Hot Cakes w/Butter, Syrup	214	500	7.9	93.9	10.3	47
Scrambled Eggs	98	180	13.2	2.5	13.0	514
Sausage	53	210	9.8	0.6	18.6	39
English Muffin w/Butter	63	186	5.0	29.5	5.3	15
Hash Brown Potatoes	55	125	1.5	14.0	7.0	7
Vanilla Shake	291	352	9.3	59.6	8.4	31
Caramel Sundae	165	361	7.0	60.8	10.0	31
Apple Pie	85	253	1.9	29.3	14.3	12
McDonaldland Cookies	67	308	4.0	49.0	10.8	10
Chocolate Chip Cookies	69	342	4.0	45.0	16.3	18
WENDY'S:						
Single Hamburger,						
Multigrain Bun	119	340	25	20	17	67
Single Hamburger, White Bun	117	350	21	27	18	65
Double Hamburger, White Bun	197	560	41	24	34	125
Bacon Cheeseburger,						
White Bun	147	460	29	23	28	65
Chicken Sandwich,						
Multigrain Bun	128	320	25	31	10	59
Kid's Meal Hamburger (2 oz)	75	220	13	11	8	20
Chili (8 oz)	256	260	21	26	8	30
French Fries, regular	98	280	4	35	14	15
Taco Salad	357	390	23	36	18	40
Frosty Dairy Dessert	243	400	8	59	14	50

Food item	Wt.	Energy	Protein	Carb.	Fat	Chol.
	grams	kcal	grams	grams	grams	mg
Hot Stuffed Baked Potatoes:						
Plain	250	250	6	52	2	tr
Sour Cream and Chives	310	460	6	53	24	15
Cheese	350	590	17	55	34	22
Chili and Cheese	400	510	22	63	20	22
Bacon and Cheese	350	570	19	57	30	22
Broccoli and Cheese	365	500	13	54	25	22
Ham and Cheese Omelette	114	250	18	6	17	450
Ham, Cheese and Mushroom Omelette	118	290	18	7	21	355
Ham, Cheese, Onion and Green Pepper Omelette	128	280	19	7	19	525
Mushroom, Onion and Green Pepper Omelette	114	210	14	7	15	460
Breakfast Sandwich	129	370	17	33	19	200
French Toast, 2 slices	135	400	11	45	19	115
Home Fries	103	360	4	37	22	20

Sources: Kentucky Fried Chicken Corp., McDonald's Corp., Wendy's International, Inc.

Nutrient analyses: Hazelton Laboratory of America, Madison, WI and U.S. Department of Agriculture *Composition of Food*, Handbook No.8.

Selected References

Aloia, John F. and others. *Diabetes, The Comprehensive Self-Management Handbook*. New York: Doubleday and Company, Inc., 1984.

Ashley, Richard and Duggal, Heidi. *Dictionary of Nutrition*. New York: St. Martin's Press, 1975.

Barnard, Dr. Christiaan and Evans, Peter. *Your Healthy Heart*. New York: McGraw-Hill Book Company, 1985.

Barness, Lewis A. "Cholesterol and Children." *Journal of the American Medical Association*, Vol. 256, No. 20, November 28, 1986, p. 2871.

Bennett, Cleaves M. *Control Your High Blood Pressure Without Drugs!* New York: Doubleday and Company, Inc., 1984.

Blair, A and Fraumeni, J.F. "Geographic Patterns of Prostate Cancer in the United States." *Journal of National Cancer Institute*, 61, 1978, pp. 1379-1384.

Carroll, K.K. and others. "Dietary Fat and Mammary Cancer." *Canadian Medical Association Journal*, 23, 1968, pp. 590-594.

Castelli, William P. and others. "Incidence of Coronary Heart Disease and Lipoprotein Cholesterol Levels, The Framingham Study." *Journal of the American Medical Association*, Vol. 256, No. 20, November 28, 1986, p. 2835.

Cohen, Leonard A. "Diet and Cancer." *Scientific American*, Vol. 257, No. 5, November 1987, pp. 42-48.

195

Correa, Pelayo. "Epidemiological Correlations Between Diet and Cancer Frequency." *Cancer Research*, Vol. 41, 1981, p. 3685.

Edelstein, Barbara. *The Underburner's Diet*. New York: Macmillan Publishing Company, 1987.

Fisher, Arthur. *The Healthy Heart*. Alexandria, Va.: Library of Health, Time-Life Books, 1981.

Gasner, Douglas and McCleary, Elliott H. *The American Medical Association Book of Heart Care*. New York: Random House, 1982.

Goor, Ron and Nancy. *Eater's Choice: A Food Lover's Guide to Lower Cholesterol*. Boston: Houghton Mifflin Company, 1987.

Hepburn, F.N. and others. "Provisional Tables on the Content of Omega-3 Fatty Acids and Other Fat Components of Selected Foods." *Journal of the American Dietetic Association*, Vol. 86, No. 6, June 1986, pp. 788-793.

Hill, P. and others. "Environmental Factors and Breast and Prostatic Cancer." *Cancer Research*, Vol. 41, September 1981, pp. 3817-3818.

Holleb, Arthur I. *The American Cancer Society Cancer Book* New York: Doubleday and Company, Inc., 1986.

Hornstra, G. and others. "Fish Oils, Prostaglandins and Arterial Thrombosis." *The Lancet*, November 17, 1979, p. 1080.

Israel, Lucien. *Conquering Cancer*. New York: Random House, Inc., 1978.

Jacobson, Michael F. and Fritschner, Sarah. *The Fast-Food Guide*. New York: Workman Publishing Company, Inc., 1986.

Kitzinger, Sheila. *The Complete Book of Pregnancy and Childbirth*. New York: Alfred A. Knopf, 1985.

Leaf, Alexander. "Fish Story." *Harvard Medical School Health Letter*, Vol. 11, No. 4, February 1986, p. 5.

Martin, Alice A. and Tenenbaum, Frances. *Diet Against Disease* Boston: Houghton Mifflin Company, 1980.

McGee, Harold. *On Food and Cooking*. New York: Charles Scribner's Sons, 1984.

Ministry of Agriculture, Fisheries and Food. *Manual of Nutrition*. London: Her Majesty's Stationery Office, 1976.

Nasset, Edmund Sigurd. *Nutrition Handbook*, Third Edition. New York: Harper and Row, 1982.

Paul, A.A. and Southgate, D.A.T. *McCance and Widdowson's The Composition of Foods*, Fourth Edition. London: Her Majesty's Stationery Office, 1978.

Paul, A.A. and Southgate, D.A.T. *First Supplement to McCance and Widdowson's The Composition of Foods*. London: Her Majesty's Stationery Office, 1980.

Phillips, R.L. "Role of Life-Style and Dietary Habits in the Risk of Cancer among Seventh-Day Adventists." *Cancer Research*, 35, 1975, pp. 3513-3522.

Royal College of Physicians of London. "Report on Obesity." *Journal of the Royal College of Physicians*, Vol. 17, 1983, pp. 5-65.

Skalka, Patricia. *The American Medical Association Guide to Health and Well-being after Fifty*. New York: Random House, revised 1984.

Tannahill, Reay. *Food in History*. New York: Stein and Day, 1973.

U.S. Department of Agriculture. *Composition of Food*, Handbook No. 8. Washington D.C., 1976.

U.S. Department of Agriculture. *Nutritive Value of American Foods*, Agriculture Handbook No. 456. Washington D.C., 1975.

U.S. Department of Agriculture. *Nutritive Value of Foods,* Home and Garden Bulletin No. 72. Washington D.C., revised 1985.

Weiner, Michael A. "Cholesterol in Foods Rich in Omega-3 Fatty Acids." *New England Journal of Medicine*, Vol. 315, No. 13, September 25, 1986, p. 833.

Whitaker, Julian M. *Reversing Heart Disease*. New York: Warner Books, Inc., 1985.

Zamula, Evelyn. "The Greenland Diet: Can Fish Oils Prevent Heart Disease?" *FDA Consumer*, Vol. 20, No. 8, October 1986, p. 6.

Index